SCREAM:

The Dark and Humorous Lessons from a Cancer Warrior

I dedicate this book to my brother Michael, a BC warrior for over 36 years. He died during COVID on September 1, 2020 at the young age of 65. Love and faith carried him every day. I wish then I had my red cape. I miss him dearly.

Acknowledgments

The journey to *Scream: The Dark and Humorous Lessons from a Cancer Warrior* started over three years ago as what I called my "little bathroom book," a little book you read instead of your cell phone while sitting on the toilet. It is written with great love to those who wonder what it's like to get the news that you have cancer and an even greater love to those who are struggling with this vicious disease. My hope is that you find inspiration through my journey and don't give up swinging.

I am grateful to my wonderful team of doctors who literally became my *team* in fighting this health battle. You've inspired my research, supported my desire for different perspectives, and gave me confidence in your knowledge. But what I love most is that you know I am the CEO.

I am grateful to all of my good friends and family members who've encouraged me to write about one of "our" stories. Some I wrote about, and some I didn't. If you are not mentioned as one of my stories, please forgive me and know that I thank you for your support.

My heart goes out to my editor, Nailah, who was given what she thought was an outline by my husband—who surprised me with a book-editing service for my 61st birthday—only to discover when she met me, it was my "finished" little bathroom book. You've encouraged me to draw out my creativity and passion from within in order to make my manuscript a better version of itself. I'm grateful that you always forgave me when I submitted drafts two hours before our weekly meetings. ☺

Speaking of gratitude, I am exceedingly grateful to my sweet children, Lily and Henry, who inspire me to live every day and literally reprimand me when I reach for sugar. I wouldn't know what to do without your daily calls. To my sweet Hannah, my stepdaughter, I am so thankful you came into my life at eight years old with such love and conviction. You three have shared my cancer journey with such laugher, tears, support, and love. You warm my heart.

Lastly, this book wouldn't have happened without Ben—my husband, my life partner. Your emotional support knows no bounds. You're at my side every day, and you're my biggest supporter. You are my red cape.

Table of Contents

My Red Cape

"Help me!"

These two words were yelled during the longest one-mile scream. But first, let's start at the beginning.

Waiting in the dugout for the inning to change, 16 years ago, as my daughter's softball coach, I received a call that changed my life. Normally I wouldn't answer my phone during a game, but it was my doctor. I felt it would be bad news from my biopsy because why else would he be calling at 6:00 pm?! "Liz," he said. "It was only a 5% chance this was cancer, and yes, you have breast cancer." I screamed inside and hid my overwhelming feelings for one more inning while putting my head back in the game. Driving home with my 10-year-old daughter and eight-year-old son in the backseat, I finally found time to myself to breakdown in my room.

The first call I made when my children were not in the room was to my husband, Ben, who was out shopping with his son for high school graduation clothes. I had to wait. *Scream!* I was overcome with emotion. Nothing anyone could say would help. Honestly, all I wanted was for someone to listen to me cry, have pity on me, and give me a hug. "It's going to be okay!" is a bullshit line because who knows. Instead, try "Hope is in the heart!" These, my friends, are the true words of encouragement to a newly diagnosed cancer victim.

The word hope has four letters, which is an indication that you cannot have hope with just *one* doctor. It takes a strategic team, family, positive friends, and a positive attitude. I didn't figure this out on day one, but lucky for me, I read Kelly A. Turner's *Radical Remission: Surviving Cancer Against All Odds*. During her dissertation, Dr. Turner discovered that there were cancer patients who actually overcame the odds of their bleak diagnosis. I realized that after my crying, screaming and self-pity, that now I had hope. I could now hunker down and pick my cancer team. It's your journey. Remember, radical remission is possible. Believe in yourself.

Back to my story...

Surgery. Thirty-eight rounds of radiation. After this, I was good to go...so I thought. Stage I, they said. But we later found out it was actually Stage II. I was scared for about five years. Then, I became complacent since I was "cancer free." Ha! I continued with my normal diet and lifestyle, which consisted of lots of stress to my body. I didn't realize then I was over-exercising: seven marathons, 46 half-marathons, and routine biking of 120-150 miles per week. Free radicals, which are both normal and good for the body, are unstable atoms that can damage cells. While free radicals can be good for the body, they can also be toxic when physical exercise becomes exhausting and atoms cannot be processed by the body. *Oxidative stress* is another term used for people like me where marathoning may have been too much for my body. Free radicals [1]may affect people differently depending on what type and what intensity you exercise.

I often reflect on this time and think this combination was fatal for me. My last marathon in Berlin, Germany, I literally felt my heart acting strange—like it was going to stop. No one spoke English as I begged for help to be taken back across the Berlin wall at mile 22. I managed to get to the finish line and knew that I was done with marathoning. It was my scariest run, but all along, I honestly struggled running distances over 10 miles. I should have listened to my body. I truly believe oxidative stress got the best of me. I realized I was running from life stressors, which became a habit. Don't get me wrong, exercise is one of the key factors in radical remission, but normal exercise is recommended, like an hour every day of walking, or running sensible miles depending on your age and body, or lifting weights, even Yoga or meditation. Again, exercise is evidence based in influencing cancer survival. But who knows about those

1 https://www.ncbi.nlm.nih.gov/pmc/articles/PMC5908316/

marathons, I guess I could cure cancer if I knew for sure. A cure for cancer…that's another story.

Fast forward to 2018, sixteen years after my first diagnosis, I was on a graduation cruise with my son and his friend. I felt a large, hard knot in my right breast. It was so big and had gotten bigger in just the last few months. With hardly any mobile service, I called my husband from the upper deck of the boat every morning. This particular morning, I explained the knot and asked him to please schedule me an appointment with my plastic surgeon right after this cruise. Thinking it was scar tissue from radiation in the implant that was in my right breast, I wasn't overly concerned; however, I had this sinking feeling. *Remember the five percent.* This percentage has always stuck in mind as it represents possibility, and not in the good way. I will always hate that number.

Without any scans, I was told that the lump was breast cancer and I needed to act quickly. After feeling the knot, the plastic surgeon told me that I needed to decide if I was going to have a double mastectomy. I was literally in shock. *You asshole! I'm here alone and driving home alone. Why would you tell me this without being absolutely sure and if you were sure, then for goodness' sake, let my oncologist tell me and Ben.* I had to sit in my car for an hour before I could safely get on the road. I didn't call anyone because I started thinking he could be wrong. I hoped he was wrong. SCREAM!!!

~

My brother was 30 when he received his first breast cancer diagnosis. His surgeons performed a radical mastectomy. Ten years later, it came back as secondary breast cancer on the same side. Keep in mind this was thirty-five years ago. Doctors weren't as knowledgeable. Technology wasn't as advanced. Online research wasn't as abundant. His doctor sent him home. No radiation. No… nothing. Just a scarred breast. I watched his struggle with cancer for thirty-five years. It was all based on traditional medicine, and his team included his one doctor. What he said is only what my brother would or would not do in his treatment. It was my brother's attitude

3

that carried him through this long up-and-down hill battle. Honestly, we fought over other things he could be doing but my brother felt like we were dealt cancer, so we should live with it and accept it. I, on the other hand, refuse to be put in that square box. I am fortunate, though, that we're related as I have his determination. (Our siblings call it meanness. Ha!)

A vibrant 57. That was my age at the time of my second diagnosis with breast cancer. The same right side. Apparently, even after thirty-eight rounds of radiation, tiny, microscopic cancer cells can survive. If I could go back in time, would I have had the mastectomy the first time? Maybe. My brother's cancer came back after a radical mastectomy on the same side as secondary breast cancer. Don't ever become complacent. The doctors told me it wasn't necessary. And I don't believe in regrets. At all.

But with this news on that day, I was alone…again. *Scream! Scream! Scream!* I had a good cry at home and then thought that he could be wrong. After all, he is only a plastic surgeon. Perhaps this is localized like the first time and requires another surgery. As it turned out, he was right, and I was wrong. Five percent again. I will always despise this number.

After several doctors' visits, a double mastectomy, and a plea with doctors for a CT scan before more surgery, I discovered the cancer had metastasized to my bones. And if you're wondering who I was with when I found out this news, the answer is no one. Ben traveled a lot and my daughters were living in Los Angeles and D.C., and my son was off at college in Chattanooga. I was sitting alone at a movie theatre when the nurse called me without asking if I was alone. She revealed that I had Stage IV cancer which had metastasized to my bones.

I drove the longest mile of my life from the movie theatre to my home. Scream! My body was literally shaking from the moment I left *Deadpool 2*, which was only 15 minutes in (and I loved the first film in the series). The nurse just blurted out this horrible devastating news and then blabbed on chirpily about her fun weekend.

Through my pain, I said to her, "Shut up! I don't give a fuck about your weekend you selfish person." That felt good. Hopefully, she learned a lesson that day to be compassionate when sharing devastating news and to always ask patients, "Are you alone?" I learned another big lesson early on in this journey, and that is you must be your own patient advocate.

I had to insist on the scan because after finding cancer in two of the four lymph nodes, my team wanted to do more surgery to check more lymph nodes. *Why?* I'm glad I held my ground because the scan revealed the shocking news, and it also revealed that I would have gotten "unnecessary" surgery. *Unnecessary surgery?* Well, that should be my choice and your choice. So, yes to the neck lift. Yes to the removal of eye wrinkles. Yes to whatever you may want to have done. *Why not?* My thinking is, if I have to die of cancer, then I want to look good until the end. And if I go into this hard-fought remission, then I still win by picking my own surgeries. Listen, I'm just saying do what makes you happy in the present. No judgment.

I digress.

Once again, I pulled in my driveway…distraught. This time, I got out, kneeled, and screamed to the top of my lungs. I'm surprised the neighbors didn't call 911. Ben was in Northern California with a dead cell phone so I couldn't reach him. (At least I thought his phone was dead.) I couldn't tell my children at that time as I would be consoling them and right then, I needed the consoling. I felt so alone. *Who would understand?* I called my brother who had cancer and whose metastasis happened the last five years of his life. I was crying so hard that he couldn't understand me.

At some point over the next several hours of nonstop screaming and crying, Ben listened to my frantic voice mails. He first called my friend Susan to share the news and ask for her help. She dropped her evening plans and came right over. She walked through the door while I was on the phone with my brother to whom he said, "I've never met her but love her like family." He knew I needed someone in person to share this bad news.

Honestly, this was my most devastating moment in my life,

and I still scream inside and out on some days. And guess what, my friends? That's okay. Screaming is most likely needed to keep you from bursting. And you know what else? In your darkest moment(s), you will discover your true friends—those that will drop everything for you. My poor husband saw so many voicemails and messages that he took a redeye home. I can only imagine what he must have felt those five hours. Remember, our caregivers also feel pain. I'll embellish this later.

~

Remember the cruise? The boys and I met Laura on day two, and we became fast friends. Being an extreme extrovert, I've always had a passion for meeting new people. For some reason, I knew Laura and I would always keep in touch. My new friend from Seattle sent me the best gift the minute she heard the news. She saw the news on Facebook. She immediately reached out to me by text with a message of love and hope. I do love Facebook for sharing news really fast. I initially shared on this social media platform to get prayers and advice, and I realized later this was not good as kind-hearted people want to tell you what to do or how to do it, and these same people did not have Stage IV cancer.

Laura, my friend from the cruise is the one who sent me the *Radical Remission* book. It is the book that I currently give to those with a new cancer diagnosis. It's the gift that keeps on giving. How amazing that a stranger can have such compassion for a new friend they just met. Another lesson learned: listen to what your friend is really saying. Maybe a cry for help that is more than just words or a quick emoji on Facebook.

I devoured the author's words. It gave me a new purpose to live, to heal, to survive, and to climb out of the grips of cancer with all my resources: my cancer team. And this is not just a traditional cancer team that is composed of only western medicine doctors. My cancer team is now composed of all kinds of doctors, my loving spouse, my children, my friends, my network, my research, and most importantly, my attitude. I hope that *my* words help *you* find your new normal. I made the decision to grab my red cape, and I'm urging you to grab yours.

Let the healing begin.

PART I: The News! Now What?

SCREAM! Throw a temper tantrum. You deserve this moment. Here's a secret, you may have a few more temper tantrums, and it's okay. I always wanted to do this anyway even when I didn't have any cancer. Every day, I decided to take a 30–40-minute nap depending on how tired I felt. I still do this till this day. I would grab the softest blanket, snuggle up, and pray myself to sleep, being grateful for everything I could think of until I dozed off. That blanket and those naps became my inspiration for the red cape. *Over the course of writing this book, my red cape has derived much more meaning. You'll see.*

This is the hardest part, my friend: accepting the reality. You will feel the pain at its very deepest level. This is okay because you'll have to decide if you want to live or go down a rabbit hole…and you don't want to choose the rabbit hole.

Scream

When my daughter had colic, I remember sitting her down in her car seat one day and then going out in the backyard for a good long scream. When my brother died, I sat on the sofa and cried so hard that it turned into a scream. Experts say that it's healthy to meditate, as it can carry you more calmly through the day and help you manage symptoms of certain medical conditions. In other words, meditation means less stress and better emotional well-being. Guess what, I believe it's just as healthy to scream. I haven't met anyone that meditated when they got the cancer news.

Honestly, until I read Dr. Turner's book, I screamed most days as I thought about pain to come, dying without ever seeing my children marry—much less grandchildren, and retiring without exploring the world with Ben. I was sad my father died, and I couldn't share my devastating Stage IV cancer news along with my fears, I was also sad that my mom had dementia and wouldn't remember the next day even if I told her. I didn't. I thought telling my parents would somehow make this all better—make it go away. What do you do? How can anyone feel your deepest personal mental pain anyway? Well, imagine someone close to you dying and then triple that pain. That's what I felt, but eventually, I decided enough was enough.

Sometimes, the thought of more cancer can create a hugging-with-fierce-crying scream that turns into happy-scream news. For example, one night shortly after my diagnosis, Ben and I were getting ready for bed and he noticed my right eye was dilated. He rushed me to the urgent care clinic. The doctor looked at me, knowing my condition, and said there is nothing we can do—it's most likely a brain tumor. We called my oncologist who said they were referring me to a specialist the next day. We cried hardcore tears that night until we fell asleep. I've never seen Ben cry like this before.

Hands and legs shaking, we walked into the optometrist's office the next day. "Did you put something in your eye?" the doctor asked a few seconds after looking at me. "Yes! My right eye was bothering me, and Ben gave me his eye drops. I only put them in my right eye," I replied. He looked annoyed at us both. "Well, of course the eye drops dilated your eye." In front of him and God, I jumped up like a pole vaulter and screamed with joy and gratitude for those damn eye drops. The optometrist didn't seem overjoyed, but he didn't have cancer. *Whew!* I dropped my red cape.

Enough with the news about illness, I don't want to go down that rabbit hole. That's not me. I want to live by the Latin aphorism, "carpe diem" every single day. Not next week. Not next month. Not next year. Every day. I choose to be present every single day that I am alive.

~

Scream! That's my advice to you. Literally Scream. In my experience, this release will allow you to feel the pain and then move forward. And friend, it's very important that you move forward. I'll be right there with you in spirit as I continue also to move forward every day. Together, with a positive healing attitude, we will begin a kickass journey of hope and healing. After you are done screaming, please grab your red cape!

Find Your Superhero

Kids love superheroes. Heck, I think we all do. Who doesn't want to be so phenomenal at something—to perhaps have superpowers?! But here's the secret to excellence, you have to put in the work. You have to put in the hours it takes to become an expert. Life gifts us with a huge brain so let's put it to good use.

No matter your favorite genre of movies or television, there's always a superhero. A superhero rarely loses, they are kind (usually cute or handsome) and they always put up a good fight. When you have cancer you need to find your superhero because you are in for the fight for your life. My children's yin and yang of movie genre really influenced my life and how I relate to a superhero.

Think about the marvel superheroes that first stared in romantic comedies: Bradley Cooper ("He's Just Not That Into You"), Chris Evans and Chris Pratt ("What's Your Number"), and Robert Downey, Jr. ("Only You"). There are so many great ones. My daughter Lily loves romantic comedies, and I realize that as an adult, she now expects her partner to be that superhero-type that she sees in her favorite films - old and new. She was so serious about her career choice that she pursued her dream to live and work in California; one of only two high school students that left Nashville and moved clear across the USA to college to study film, business (and Spanish). Her dad and I influenced both of our children's love of travel. Lily was a pro traveler at the age of one.

After chasing that dream and fighting the woos of Hollywood, she is now working in television at Sony. Her boyfriend recently shared his engagement plans and what he thought would be the perfect engagement, and I laughed. "You want to ask my daughter to marry you? Watch a romantic comedy and come back to me with your idea." He ended up proposing in Central Park on Bow Bridge. A super Rom Com moment. Now that's the spirit. P.S. I was lucky he made me and her dad part of this plan. This I did get to see and I'll be forever grateful to Justin.

My son Henry is quite the opposite. He is an extreme introvert and loves action movies—especially the Marvel ones (those same guys that were the love heroes in the romantic comedies). I realize that his perception of a superhero was also impacted by this favorite movie genre. Most superheroes are introverts when you think about it. They save the world, but then go back to their quiet life.

One of Henry's favorite toys as well as movies (you always get ripped off as a parent when they make the superhero toy), were the Power Rangers. Remember those initial five teenagers that would morph into a Power Ranger with some special power to combat evil. Brilliant. This influenced, at the time, so many little boys and I'm sure girls (just not mine). Halloween one year all I saw were little Power Rangers. They are always there for you when needed, but then disappear back to normal. Behind the scenes they are plotting their brilliance.

Find your superhero. Mine—thanks to my children—is a combination of the two genres that they love. I find compassion in the romantic comedies and determination in the action movies. Are you wondering who my super hero is? It's Wonder Woman. She is the God of the hunt, the moon and nature from Roman mythology. She never ages and has superhuman strength. She is both action and romance. Her superpowers are in alignment with both genres of movies. Plus, she wears a cape.

There's a side of me that seems to always root for the underdog, surprise an elderly person with a free lunch, donate to a new organization. The other side of me will fight like a lion (I'm a Leo) for my loved ones. And that fight is where I am now—I won't stop striving for healing. You shouldn't either. A cancer victim needs that superhuman strength. Find your superhero.

You are embarking on a kick-ass journey. Put on that red cape, my friend. Gently put it down to have your temper tantrum, as needed, then put it the F back on. Every day, imagine yourself as a superhero with a supernatural belief that you can conquer this journey. You are stronger and smarter than you think, and you look damn good in that red cape.

Call a Friend

Call only the friend that will make you laugh in your darkest moment. You will find not all friends are your true friends. Of course, when you get this news, you'll just want to scream it to every friend as if this might make it go away - or just saying it out loud more will finally make it real. It's crazy. It's intolerable. It's lonely. It's dark. It's not fucking fair.

Who was your first "I have cancer" call? Mine, the second time around with Stage IV cancer news, was to Ben. Remember his dead cell phone that I thought was turned off? I left around 20 voicemails thinking he would eventually call me, but I appreciate that he eventually checked his voicemail and asked my friend, Susan, could she help. She said she dropped everything to head to our home. When she walked through my door, she grabbed me, and we fell into a chair. "Oh, honey!" She literally held me like a baby and we both cried until I started laughing because I couldn't breathe. We talked about life and death over a glass of wine and the chicken pot pie I forgot that I had made (a bit later that evening she laughed that she asked me for food considering the situation). Finally, Susan decided it was late and she was staying over. She slept in the same bed to "watch me." Of course she asked for pajamas, and not just any pajamas, but the brand name PJ Savage pajamas. They are the best. Ha! Susan was that friend that was there for me and that made me laugh in my darkest moment.

After the first call, I made many calls the next day to other friends. Warning: you must be prepared for that awkward silence and the awkward responses because not everyone knows what to say. It's okay. Not everyone is equipped to deal with cancer. Obviously, I wasn't okay, and I learned that "the news" touches deep in everyone's soul no matter how they verbally express themselves.

When my brother shared his news at 30 years old, I was only 24. Wasn't this a woman's disease? He was calm and never wanted anyone to worry about him. When I shared my news with him—the second time around—after I calmed down, he told me that he never had anyone to talk to about this journey that would really understand. He wasn't one to share his feelings. And at that moment, I realized that I hadn't really been a true friend or loving sister to him. From that day forward, we spoke every single day. Some days it was about cancer, most often it was not.

The point of this story is to call a friend every day. No texting, but real honest-to-goodness calls. Gratitude will be felt simultaneously. You'll never know what is going on in someone's life that day and how a simple conversation will uplift spirits.

Cancer is a moment of reality - whom you can depend on now and through your journey. Cry together, but end your tears with laughter, very tight hugs, a glass of red wine or perhaps a valium or gummy to sleep, and then place that red cape gently beside your bed.

I Scream, Now You Scream

You will probably tell your family the news first. This can be as hard as hearing the damn news. Your children will be terrified, and if they're under the age of 25, they may think, "Will this happen to me, too?" or "Wait, I can't lose you." Nevertheless, they will also be at a deep personal loss for words. That was okay with me because no words were needed, just hugs and tears. I've always had a very close relationship with Lily and Henry, and you know what I love about them as we're almost four years into this—they treat me the same. I have to even use the C-card a.k.a. the cancer card as I like to say. It's one of the only times I get to use this ugly word for good to get my children's attention sometimes. This means I've done my job and in their own way, they have accepted our journey. For now.

I can only wish I had parents I could've shared this horrible painful news with. And siblings? They are different flowers from the same garden. My siblings are not the best at sharing their feelings nor having the comforting words that you may think being family. "You'll be fine." "Oh no!" "I'm so sorry." It's family; we don't choose them, but we love the hell out of them.

I knew I wouldn't get the support I desired from my siblings even before calling them. We grew up with an alcoholic father and a mother who struggled with four children while dealing with my father's addiction. We learned to survive, to hide during the fighting, to leave in the middle of the night, to fall asleep during school, and to put on a front with our friends because they came from what seemed like a normal family. I never invited friends to my drama house because it would have made the news at school. Whispers, laughter, stink eyes…it's still there today. We call it judgment as adults. This struggle made us closer in ways no one else could understand and stronger individuals; however, you couldn't meet four more different siblings. Interestingly enough, none of us grew up as alcoholics or smokers. I may take a pot gummy to sleep but I don't smoke it. Still, don't tell my mom because this she might not forget. ☺

When my dad was dying, I drove to Atlanta from Nashville, mindlessly grinding my teeth, thinking about what I wanted to say to this man who had gone through so much pain himself. How did his life influence mine?! At the side of his bed, it was hard seeing his blue eyes that had gone grey from lack of oxygen. I started spilling my guts at the tremendous love and value he brought to my life, with my family in the room. Oh wait, no…they had all left. I thought they were listening and would then say their own words but as usual, they disappeared. I think they were embarrassed to hear my heartfelt words to our Dad. We didn't grow up sharing our feelings. In fact, all my brothers and sisters could say when I said I had cancer was, "You'll be okay." Fuck. And you know what? I am okay. It took a minute and somewhere along the way, I've learned to share my feelings, and most of the time they're good.

By the way, that darn grinding on my drive to Atlanta haunted me a week later at my daughter's basketball game. I was talking to a friend in the stands, and my front tooth popped out of my mouth and landed on the court during the game. My friend said, "Was that your tooth?" I was mortified. No joke. I'm sure my dad was smiling. I called my sister as I knew she would wet her pants laughing which would make me laugh even harder. I loved to make her laugh and to this day we share so much laugher.

Show your family your fighting spirit, your superhero attitude, and of course, your red cape. It's okay to scream together, as a family, because perhaps this sets the stage for them to be a part of your cancer team. Perhaps this will help them understand how it feels to not only hear these words, but to have to live and fight this diagnosis. You are now their superhero and they are watching and counting on you. It's okay to share your red cape.

Write Down Your Feelings

I call BS on this one for now. I say this because I feel that you first have to come to grips with your diagnosis before even assessing your feelings. That's like telling me to meditate after I got the news. No, thank you. I think I'd rather scream. But to each his own. Scream or do what you need to do to help you feel the pain, and then get the hell up and take control of your situation. I promise it's not easy and some days it feels unbearable. I mean on a travel day, I can't poop and it's the most miserable day or days, but then I finally do, and it feels all better.

Facebook. It seems these days that people use this social media platform as the main platform for their feelings. This is tricky. I agree that it's wise to use social media to ask for prayers. As the adage states, "It takes a village…" That said, I'll take all the villages when it comes to prayers. But then I ask myself, "Am I good enough for God to heal me or sweet enough?" This is the biggest worry. Ha! Get your mind and faith right and say yes I can heal - "all things are possible for those that believe." Don't quote me as I didn't look up the bible verse but how I remember this one. I do believe. I also think it's wise to stay away from politics on social media because you don't need this stress. Think about politics and how divisive it is when you hear people arguing in person. For the most part, people are not going to change their opinion about an issue based off someone's Facebook post. It only can incite bad feelings or thoughts because you want to say something but know it will start a war of words. Stress. My advice is to ignore the post. Don't respond. Unfollow a politically motivated person. Move on for your health.

I use Facebook because I love seeing what's going on in my family and friends' lives. The only reason I opened an account was because I wanted details on my 20-year high school reunion. I wanted to make sure I recognized everyone when I saw them in person. It mostly worked, but name tags would've worked better. Most of my friends are longtime high school friends that, ironically, never knew my true life's story. These same friends today, with which I've reconnected with through Facebook, have become real friends. They are my prayer warriors. This is *one* of my villages. I give a shout out to all my Rockdale County High School friends.

You can learn a lot about people from their posts. I became Facebook friends with a lady from a group where I volunteered as a fitness trainer. She is pure sunshine. I look forward to her daily "good mornings," her posts about her children, her beautiful prayers, and her uplifting spirit. In all these years, she has never posted one single negative post about anything. Seriously, let me know if you need this kind of Facebook friend because she'll let you in. Thanks, Lawanda.

If you often come across negative and/or nasty posts, my advice is to unfollow or unfriend. Kick stress to the curb so you can get to your healing. Pray first. Share your anger, your fear, and your plan to heal? Not there yet? Get your game on, my friend. You can and you must. Feelings will ebb and flow, and it's okay because even without cancer, this happens in life anyway. Was Rome built in a day? No. It took me getting into my healing journey before I could face this reality called cancer and write. This does take a minute, but your red cape will be waiting for you. Speaking of time, it took me well over a year to even start writing this book. Give yourself grace, and let your words flow when you're ready.

PART II: Build Your Team

This is the beginning of a very radical journey, or not. I reached beyond traditional medicine with a functional oncologist who believes in combining both western and eastern medicine. You can find him in Radical Remission: Surviving Cancer Against all Odds. It really does take a village. Ben and I have talked to doctors in England, Germany, and Mexico. No consultations, just conversations. The decision is yours. Hope is the magic word that I keep on the tip of my tongue every day. Hope is often misunderstood. People tend to think that it is simply passive wishful thinking, I hope something will happen, but I'm not going to do anything about it. This is indeed the opposite of real hope, which requires action and engagement. Hunker down, my friend, of course with that red cape over your shoulders.

Doctors: The Good, the Bad, the Ugly

Doctors, they are not God. He is the Master Healer. Get more than one opinion. And for goodness' sake, throw cancer spittle on them if they tell you to eat whatever you want, especially sugar. Then run. Most importantly, do not let them give you statistics. People tend to count down their days when this is the news.

My first oncologist made us wait two hours, and then walked into the room with no apologies for the wait. She proceeded to tell me I can eat all the sugar I wanted and even encouraged it. We basically told her to pack sand and Ben and I walked out. Not all doctors are created equal, and you must advocate for yourself. We are all terrified to talk about our plan, but damnit, a doctor like this is not the doctor I want to make my plan.

In a SugarAidsCancerGrowth[2] article, there are scholarly references to this enemy called sugar. It took me about two weeks honestly to give up simple sugars. At first, I felt tired and lethargic and even lost weight over those two weeks, but I discovered a newfound healthy energy. This may or may not be the same for you, but please research the meaning of simple sugars and act accordingly. I still eat all berries, including pineapple and green apples (which have less sugar) every day. I always chose the morning because I know I will walk off those calories. These fruits, as sugars, respond differently on tumors than simple sugars. I'll share more about this later. A cheat day every now and then is fine as long as you can take that urge and "turn it back off." The point is, find a doctor that supports your beliefs.

My current oncologist is an amazing lady. She supports my decision to also have a functional medicine oncologist. I promised her no hiding what I've decided to include in my journey. Sometimes her eyebrows raise, especially when I told her about scorpion venom,

2 https://dss.ncf.edu/cancerwiki/index.php/ SugarAidsCancer-Growth

but always with a big smile. Her answer is Stage IV cancers take more than just traditional medicine. This is when I knew I found the right doctor. Mind you, she never offers more than this, but she supports my right to more. Most importantly, she never gives statistics. One day, I asked her if she has any patients exactly like me that are still alive after 10 years and she said yes. I didn't ask beyond this because at the time, this Stage IV was all new to me and ten years was sounding promising.

~

Scans are scary. Every three to four months, you wait for the news…all news. I refuse to look at my health portal which has the results posted long before I see my oncologist. I wait two days later. I don't want to read anything that could possibly be bad and panic. I play this game: I wait until she walks in the door and read her face and body language. "Your scans are…great." My oncologist, Ben, and I do a little cheer for those results. Before COVID, we hugged. We discuss anything new or on the horizon, which sadly, there is still nothing for my cancer going on four years. We talk about our families and planned travel. I love her and feel confident I chose the right traditional oncologist. Thanks, Dr. Abramson.

My dermatologist/cosmetologist has become a special friend over our years together. A Harvard trained doctor who moved to the South and is the most humble doctor I've ever met. I took advantage of him being new, and also his staff if I had to wait too long. I would leave my room and go find him to remind him that my time also was valuable. This became a joke at his office. When he found out about my cancer metastasis, he walked into my appointment and without saying a word gave me the biggest hug. I cried. Since that day, he has followed my journey on my health portal as he is a Vanderbilt University Medical Center doctor. When his brother experienced cancer, guess what? I gifted him a copy of *Radical Remission*. There are not many doctors I look forward to seeing, but he is on the top of my list. There is not a visit that we don't laugh and quickly catch up on our lives. Thanks, Dr. Stebbins.

When I devoured *Radical Remission*, it led me to whom is now my functional medicine oncologist. He used to be at Sloan Kettering Cancer Center in NYC for 10 years. Ben and I flew to NYC to meet with him in person once. Ben is the smartest person I know, yet he told me, "Liz, this is the smartest person I have met in my life." He's not great with the warm and fuzzy but who cares, he had a plan. To this day, I meet with him after every scan on Zoom. We cover all my supplements (five from him to boost my immune system, along with the many others that I researched and he approved) and we discuss non-traditional methods to beat this cancer. To date, I haven't decided to pursue any of these other methods. Why? I think because as all my doctors say I'm on a winning horse. However, I have my options ready and waiting and that in and of itself brings me peace. A secret: your homework is never done. Thanks, my special Dr. Chang.

I must give a shout out to Dr. John Anderson. He is my primary care physician, our family's hero. Long before COVID, he made sure not to expose me to sick patients. He understood the fear of walking into a waiting room with Stage IV cancer or any cancer really. He decided to give me his cell phone number and his back office number which I do not misuse. This assures me that I will skip the waiting room and get in faster to see him if needed, or that I may not even need to come in and he can answer me by cell phone. I respect that he has put me on a pedestal and has gifted me with no fear to see my doctor. Again, it's about your team. Choose wisely.

All cancers and all doctors are not created equal. All good things come to those who work hard, and that red cape gives you superpowers when needed.

Research, read, don't settle for a quack. This is your decision, your interview, and your journey. If you get scared or intimidated, have a moment, grab your red cape, and then jump back in and find your team.

Radical Remission

Buy it, read it, read it again. This book will bring light to the darkness by inspiring you with the many remission stories of those who've once suffered from various stages of cancer. I included it in this section because it has been a part of my team. If it weren't for this book, I wouldn't have known where to begin. Dr. Tracy A. Kelly Turner's *Radical Remission: Surviving Cancer Against All Odds* got me started on my journey after that very dark day of hearing "you have Stage IV cancer." And it continues today after more than three years. Even today, I pick up the book to reread in case I've missed something. It's kind of like a great movie you love and decide to watch it again and exclaim, "Oh, I didn't see that the first time."

I found my functional medical oncologist and my holistic therapist in this book. I found another cancer survivor that wrote about beating cancer and part of his journey included juicing recipes. I swear they should send a red cape with this book. You don't hear about these testimonials because how would the medical world make millions more if we could actually cure cancer? Hmm.

Cancer has been cured over and over, and every time stripped away from the beautiful doctor that found a cure by the American Medical Association, and the Food and Drug Administration viciously. For my film lovers, there's an informative series that you can stream called "The Truth About Cancer." It's a tad complicated to decipher all the information out there; however, it exposes a lot of untold truths about cancer. There is also a self-titled book and a website with lots of information that is outside the scope of western medicine with lots of doctor conversations from all over the world.

It is important to not give up hope and to believe that you can be one of the radical remission survivors that we will read about one day.

Cancer Groups

Honestly, cancer groups in person are not for me. To each his own. Positive, fun, energetic groups of friends are what I choose to do instead. I can't do negativity because it takes the sunshine out of my day and the stars out of the sky. I love both my sunshine and my stars. For me, the cancer groups that I initially tried to attend in person, I found the people to be whiny, depressing and accepting of their demise. Not for me, I choose positivity. The mind is very strong and has a lot of control over your health. No crybabies,

Don't get me wrong, there is a time and place for tears and screams. For me, it is with my closest friends and Ben. For me, I feel most supported when someone can just listen and then give me a fierce hug and perhaps compassionate tears.

You may have friends and want to start your own cancer group. Do what works for you. I don't have a group of cancer friends per se, but when I come across others who have been diagnosed, I make sure to send them an uplifting note and my favorite book. We may or may not follow each other on Facebook after this, however, I encourage anyone and everyone to have hope and to get busy with your healing journey.

I knew these types of traditional in-person cancer groups were not for me after a few visits. You have to decide what type of journey is right for you. Keep yourself healthy, happy, and strong for your journey. Remember, you have your red cape, and you are not a babysitter. You are a product of your team and an example of positivity.

The Exception

There is one exception to the previous chapter, and that is positive Facebook support groups—cancer groups that share their remission stories and make you check your ego and politics at the door. If all the angry political people on both sides had cancer, they might redirect their attention to what really matters—like allowing a cure for cancer, instead of more pharmaceutical money. Just saying.

I follow a Facebook group called Jane McLelland Off Label Drugs for Cancer. While I thought Jane's book was overly complicated, her cancer group is awesome. I follow this group to see if there is anyone out there like me that is beating cancer in a different way. If I think they are, I research the heck out of what they are taking that I'm not, and then run it by my functional oncologist, Dr. Chang. A few others groups that I like are Cancer Immunotherapy, Curt Michael Graydon - Artemisinin, Fenbendazole, Cancer/Health Protocols, and The Sacred Plant. Now keep in mind that I read these, I don't always act on everything I read, but it does make me ask questions and consider alternatives. Mostly, these groups give me hope.

Once a day, I sit and scroll Facebook making sure I haven't missed a birthday or a special event in a friend's life. My brother-in-law has something like 2,000 friends. He grew up in our small town, but my sister and I tease him that he cannot possibly know all those people. He's one of those guys that never ever meets a stranger. You actually may be on his friend list. ☺

I've discovered that people who live life with love and kindness make me the most happy when I'm scrolling. They share fun stories, family or travel moments and in the case of the cancer stories I follow, they post to help each other by identifying what has or has not worked for them. No one attacks them or their decision about their cancer journey. In fact, most respond with respect and love for another cancer victim. Love for one another really conquers all. It's just that simple.

PART III: Educate Yourself

When I say educate yourself, I'm not referring to higher education. I'm earnestly talking about cancer education for your specific cancer. Do you know the details of your specific cancer? Could you explain it to someone else? Do you have access to all your history, your diagnosis, and your exact tests for your exact type of cancer? For instance, all breast cancers are not the same as most non-cancer people don't realize. I'll give a shout out to Vanderbilt as I can log in and see it all, share it all. By the way, I do this with my team. No secrets, everyone knows. A good book with true survivors of your diagnosis is also a must. Don't scan, R- E-A-D. Cover your legs with that red cape, curl up, and read.

Steady Eddie: Research, Read, Read, Read

Spend every other day researching everything you can about what may be out there for your type of cancer - trials, medicine, non-traditional healing and further researching what you may have read in a book about cancer in general, Take notes, makes calls - I have talked to doctors all over the world. Always keep in mind that there is a lot of "fake news" out there but also a lot of really good stuff. I'll mention this again, it is important to make sure that you DO NOT look at statistics. I put this right up there with fake news as every person is different. Get your mind and body in check as you start this part of your journey,

Evidence based research is great, but so are real stories of radical remission. I will be honest that you must take a vacation—albeit a short one—from your research in order not to burn out and give up. Never ever give up that red cape my friend.

Each article you read may lead you to another and another article.

Perhaps there is a doctor treating only *your* stage of cancer. Well, reach out to them by email, Skype, or WhatsApp. No one is going to do this work for you. Bury yourself in that red cape and get busy. I have spoken to doctors in other countries by WhatsApp. The more you listen, really listen, the better your ability to make decisions for yourself. Have another pair of trustworthy ears with you if you are talking to a new doctor. Take notes. Ask questions. Don't be afraid of the doctors because they are still learning about cancer, too. The doctors I researched and spoke with were kind to share what is and what is not available both in their countries and ours.

I want to expand on "The Truth About Cancer." In the Eastern part of the world, a simple spice called curcumin is added to everything. It fights inflammation and if you google curcumin and cancer, you will see the amazing reasons it's in my diet. Simple oils, like frankincense—remember it was the first gift given to baby Jesus by the wise men— has many useful properties for cancer.

Dr. Josh Ax is one of the American doctors in this streaming series and he guides you on the proper oil use as well as supplemental advice.

His mother battled cancer two times. The first time she did only traditional medicine and was so sick from chemo. As Dr. Ax said, she aged 20 years both physically and mentally. Her cancer came back nine years later and this time, Dr. Ax took her down the natural path[3]. He was determined not to see her suffer anymore, and she was willing to take this chance. She is now cancer free and thriving.

Funny story, I was walking in my old neighborhood one day and realized that my neighbor three houses down was Dr. Ax. He was always on his phone walking and of course who interrupts him but me while I was also out walking. I was so excited that this incredible person was my neighbor. I think he thought I was stalking him as I continued to see him while I was out walking after that every day. He moved six months later. Oh well, I still follow him and buy products from his website. I'm sure there is an alert by my name.

I'm combining functional with traditional medicine. Honestly, the only traditional medicines offered to me were Ibrance and Letrozol. Ibrance is not even a chemo pill but boy does it mess with your immune system. Nonetheless, it works for now. Letrozol is an estrogen blocker. I was too far gone to receive liquid chemo. You know, the one where you have a port and go every other week or two. This is only for those who can hopefully beat wherever the cancer has spread. By the way, it was very important for me not to look at the side effects of either one of these pills. This can actually cause those side effects. Mind over matter remember. Ben read them just in case, but to this day, we've never talked about them.

With my diagnosis in mind, I knew I better get busy and do more research if I wanted to outsmart this cancer. There is hope but you have to go find it yourself. Make sure your cape is not covering your eyes or ears.

---

3 https://draxe.com/health/10-natural- cancer-treatments-hidden-cures/.

Know it All, Share it All

As the African proverb puts it, "If you think you're too small to make a difference, you haven't spent the night with a mosquito." The mosquito makes a difference in an annoying way, but the principle is the same. One person can stop a great injustice. One person can be a voice for truth. One person's kindness can save a life. One person can help another with cancer. Each person matters.

Share your findings, your experiences, your frustrations and how you overcame them, your desires, and your beliefs every single day to heal. Most importantly, pray for yourself and each other. Cancer doesn't discriminate and neither does God.

This is the time to be a know-it-all. This is the time to take care of yourself, share your news, and help others who are struggling. Your purpose is you and those closest to you. Find out your specific cancer, your pathway, and your mutation, and then research again.

I have a friend named Boo who I walk with weekly. I showed her a six-mile walk and she showed me how to increase my walking pace to an average of a 16-minute mile. A lot of people run a 16-minute mile at my age. No consideration that I have cancer. Why? Because I look and feel healthy, and she knows I want to be treated like her friend—not her cancer friend. Although this may be a good time to use the C-card to slow our pace.

Boo and I talk about everything. She's my only friend with whom I can talk politics and religion and not want to slap each other afterwards. We look forward to every single walk and both of us will move mountains to make it happen.

It's a good thing the reality TV show "The Amazing Race" stopped filming because Boo and I decided that we would've definitely won the competition. We were two old ladies that would've used our Southern charm to oust our competitors. Both in agreement, Boo would've jumped out of the plane while I waited for her in the raft to rescue her and while she skydived off the cliff, I would cheer her on from the bottom as her partner. However, I would've had to eat the worms while she watched with a barf bag close by. Almost every time we walked, we plotted our "The Amazing Race" victory.

Boo makes me feel like a hero about my health and brags about me to her family and friends. I didn't know how much she bragged about me until I attended her grandson's first birthday party and was greeted by a barrage of "I've wanted to meet you," "I've heard about you," and "What do you think about this?" I remember smiling inside thinking I can even help healthy people possibly avoid cancer or other health problems. Not one person treated me with pity. It was the baby's birthday, but secretly, it was unknowingly my day to shine. Thanks, Boo.

~

My sister has a good friend whose husband is suffering from cancer and is on constant liquid chemo, an immune killer for sure. I happen to be friends with her on Facebook. In my little hometown, we all know our siblings' friends and family. When I read this horrible news about him, I reached out to my sister's friend via messenger and shared with her the responsibility to go beyond traditional medicine while making their own decision on what might work for her husband. She now shares her findings with me. It's amazing. Without knowing that I had already reached out to her, my sister one day told her friend to talk to me because I am always researching. Her friend said, "Oh, we've been communicating for a long time now." Ha! Thanks, Theresa.

Plug in your mutation, and Shazam! The red cape is on, baby!

We are all in this together.

Your Immune System

There is much evidence that supports how much your immune system will be fighting against the chemo/radiation. Your immune system is your best friend forever (BFF), especially now. All BFF can act out, and your immune system is no different. Therefore, you should constantly have to monitor this part of your health with your blood labs and make adjustments. Read and digest what is good for your immune system based on your specific type of cancer.

Before my scheduled labs, I ask my doctor every single time to check my Vitamin D level and my Iron level. My functional medicine oncologist said that quite often a chemo patient may have depleted iron levels[4]. So many times I'll talk to cancer friends who are so incredible tired they can't simply walk to the mailbox. My brother was one of those iron-depleted people, yet his doctor would not offer him iron. The result is iron deficient anemia[5] which lowers the odds of survival in cancer patients.

However, most doctors will not offer you an iron supplement. Why? They were not trained in supplements, nutrition, or exercise. Go look at their curriculum; they spend less than one day out of their career on all of these subjects. My brother's doctor didn't believe in supplements other than Vitamin D—eventually. Vitamin D3 [6]is what your body produces and should be taken with vitamin K2. Even though I watched him go from a healthy cancer patient to a very sick one, he was the strongest cancer fighter I knew in attitude and hard-headedness. I'm glad we are alike in that way. I miss him every day, and I will continue this fight for us both until I see him again.

I digress.

---

4 https://www.ncbi.nlm.nih.gov/pmc/articles/PMC5119669/
5 https://www.everydayhealth.com/hs/iron-deficiency-anemia/cancer/
6 https://www.mercola.com/article/vitamin-d-resources.htm

Moving on, most people are depleted of Vitamin D3, and when you have cancer you need a higher normal level than non-cancer people. In fact, your optimum Vitamin D3 level should be in between 60-80, if you have cancer. Unfortunately, most people don't realize their body is low on Vitamin D3 unless they request their doctor to specially check their level. Always ask. Most doctors don't know squat about vitamins because they don't make any money from vitamins. Most often a doctor will tell a cancer patient that a level of 20-35 is good. It's not! They know it's important now but are still uneducated about the proper levels, especially for people like us fighting cancer. I was taking this long before some doctors finally understood the importance.

Remember, your nutrition and supplements are more important now than ever. I'm not talking cakes and cookies people. Remember that old guy a.k.a. Hippocrates who said, "Let food be thy medicine and medicine be thy food." It still applies today However, sometimes we need more than just the food, especially when you are fighting cancer I'm now taking close to 30 supplements in the a.m. and nearly 12 in the p.m. Each one has a purpose that I have researched and that has been approved by my functional oncologist.

It's important to make conscious decisions about what to eat, what to smell, and even what you are touching as these too can affect your immune system. For instance, there are safer versions of cleaning supplies. Honestly, would you swallow a cup of Clorox? When you are cleaning you are ingesting those smells, those cancerous chemicals. Try natural cleaning products, which will also benefit your family and animals. There are enough environmental toxins out of our control but this, my red cape friend, is all on you.

Watching what I eat and which products I choose for my home and body reveal the bigger me that wants to live, and it can do the same for you. Let's make better choices so we can be one of those radical remission people.

Drop that red cape and open those supplements—the ones that are right for you and throw out those nasty chemicals.

PART IV: Inspiring Friends and Family

Dealing with family and friends can be tricky. Some of your friends will hide—they won't know what to say. Some of your friends will say too much, and others will judge what you are doing. It's common. But my advice is to let go of the negative friends in your life—the ones that make you feel exhausted or stressed after a visit. Let go of the "friends" that say mean things to you even if it is a family member. Let go of these people as they are toxic. If you don't have the strength to do this, then get help from a holistic therapist. They will help you find that needed peace and strength that you need to heal. Let go and move on. It's your journey and you are in the fight for your life.

Live Loud

Don't forget to breathe deeply and do something with a friend or family member every day. A call, a lunch, or a walk or in my case and now pickle ball. If no laughter or no fun, then don't call that person again (at least you may have gotten in a walk). Put that name inside your red cape as a reminder to mark them off your list. You need to live with love, support, and no judgment every day in every way.

As we get older and perhaps do not live in a retirement community or do not attend church in person (due to yet another COVID outbreak), it becomes hard to have daily in-person interactions. Some introverts don't mind, but this extrovert needs that social time every day. I find that my friends are now at their "other" home, scared to socialize because of COVID, or they're just busy with their own extended families. As for me, when I'm in Nashville, I go for walks every single day. While walking I call a family member or friend and if no one is available, I listen to a book on Audible.

I have college students that still check on me and I try to get them all together for social time. This is good for all of us as they didn't all know each other from class. My son's friends, all now 24 years old and older, love to visit our home as we are big game players and I'm a pretty good cook. They are kind to include Ben and me for part of the evening. Young people keep you young. It's fun to hear their perspective on current events going on in our crazy world. Lately, I have been struggling with living in Nashville due to how much I love our retirement community in Utah. I am an extreme extrovert.

I'm so fortunate that God blessed us with a new home in Utah, where I learned to play pickle ball. I met just one friend, Monica, on my first pickle ball day. The most kind, compassionate person to every stranger she meets. She invited me to her home for social hour that evening, which is very popular in our neighborhood, and she introduced Ben and me to many new friends. When I had my first social party, it was Monica who invited all my guests. Now, I have my own guest lists. They all feel like family. More friends. More pickle ball. Many fun social hours. Many e-bike rides. Lots of hiking and the most laughter and fun I've had in years.

There is not a day that goes by in our Utah neighborhood where you are not surrounded with friends. Someone is always hosting a happy hour where we all bring an appetizer and just like fun old people, we hang out from 5:30 pm to 8:30 pm so we can hurry home, get to bed early only to wake up and meet at the pickle ball courts at 7:00 am. Ha!

One of my favorite neighbors, Warren, literally will stand up, if he and his wife Cindy are hosting a social hour and say, "It's 8:30. Time to leave." Recently, I was at another social hour at another neighbor's home and noticed the time was 9:15 pm and Warren was still there. We all had a chuckle. By the way, I have to give a shout out to Warren Driggs and his incredible books about being a Mormon and then his decision not to be a Mormon. What a humorous and enlightening journey to those of us who don't understand this faith. Seriously, his three books are great reads.

What an incredible place to live: Utah. I call this neighborhood Candy Land because I never realized how important in-person socialization is at all ages. Others in our neighborhood think of our neighborhood as the movie "Cocoon." I'll let you watch that movie. Either way, it's a high energy environment for a bunch of old folks.

In Dan Buettner's book, *Blue Zones*, the National Geographic Explorer shares stories of people who live the longest and happiest with the lowest disease burden. One of the principles mentioned is "keep family first, pick the right tribe (social), and belong (faith in person)." If you want to live longer and better this is a great book. There are now communities everywhere that are "Blue Zones." These Blue Zones are making a difference across communities. I think Dan should visit my neighborhood in Utah.

Back to living loud. I do feel my best and love my life the most when I'm in Utah. I feel like a million bucks. Only a few ladies here know about my cancer, so there's no judgment and no looks. Just sheer fun. Thank you, Monica. I'm sure one day they will all be shocked to hear my news, but for now, I leave my red cape, and go on with my day. But guess what, it's there always when I come home tired and ready for my afternoon nap. I always take that nap, especially after all this activity. So seize your day and have some fun.

Laugh Often

Find humor in your situation. My brother-in-law Mike thinks it's strange that I'm writing and talking at my memorial. I figure everyone will be so upset that I would get cheated on a proper service. My celebration of life will be because I lived. My only regrets will be leaving my children and Ben. I will be cremated and put in a necklace that my hubby will wear around his neck so I can spy on him. Ha!

I will suggest my children take their part of me on a journey together of my choosing, and my select friends to take their part of me to our favorite place together. I'm not yet finished writing my memorial service but I think it's important for everyone - cancer or not - to write your own service.

My ex-husband—whose name is also Ben (I know… convenient)—always saw the importance in travel. And so did I. He made sure Lily and Henry saw every national park while I made sure they saw many beaches, many times with school friends and their moms. We even had beach names. Mine was Sunny.

My favorite trips became the ones that I took every year with Lily: our mother-daughter trip. Every year from first grade to her senior year of high school, we would piggy back off Ben's company trip to New York. He would leave the last day and we would come in and stay for the weekend. This was always the week after they lit the giant Rockefeller Christmas Tree. These are all fond memories that I think about often while laughing out loud. For example, one time Lily and I had been window shopping on Fifth Avenue and decided to walk into a shop. The attendant came up and said did you know you have bird poop all down the back of your black coat? Lily was crying laughing as she knew and didn't tell me.

Have you ever smelled those nasty peanuts cooking on the cart in NYC? Lily had to have a bag. We bought it and she only ate half and left the other ones on the desk in our room. Since it was stuffy and hot inside, I opened a window so we could get some fresh air that night. Mind you, I get up in the dark and read by a book light to wait for Lily to wake. This day we were leaving and as we were getting in the cab, the valet guy says to us "did you remember your plugs?" Of course I had left mine and ran back to retrieve it. To my surprise it was chewed to pieces and then it occurred to me. We had RATS. Giant NYC ones that had come down from the roof to that peanut smell. Most likely chewing away on my cord while I was reading in the dark. Never open your window in NYC.

These trips and memories are priceless. What I love most about their Dad is he is exactly the same when it comes to spending travel time with our children. Call it an abundance of love wanting to spend special time with your children. Sometimes it drives Lily and Henry crazy. Wait until they have their own children.

My son Henry and I have our own special journeys. While they were all great, there are two that stand out thus far. We had traveled to England. I had rented a flat, as they say, in Covent Garden. We were dropped off at the flat at 8:00 a.m. London time sleep deprived. After walking up the steepest 30 stairs I've ever seen, we discovered the flat had a very narrow spiral staircase that led to our bedrooms—one that would not accommodate our luggage so we lived out of our luggage downstairs. We were two floors above an Italian restaurant and at first the smell was wonderful but after a day we realized it was the only thing we could smell. I honestly can still smell that Italian restaurant. Our first day here, Henry realized that he had left his wallet on the airplane. Can you believe it was turned in and waiting for us a week later on our return home.

On this same trip, we did a tour to Paris. The guide was not happy when at the Eiffel Tower I told her we decided we were staying in Paris. Another spontaneous decision. Did I say we walked down the Eiffel Tower—both afraid of heights?! One day after we left, Paris had a bombing. I knew it was a possibility but why not just live in the moment because who knows, you may get cancer.

Our trip to Canada was all about Henry. He loves trains and outdoor adventure. We took the Canadian train from Vancouver and had several stops along the way to finally end in Banff. This meant we spent one night on the train. My first time to sleep on a train. The room was so tiny, but the windows were huge. I asked Henry could we leave the shades open to sleep as I was claustrophobic. Of course he said yes. He was on the top bunk, me on the bottom. Deep in sleep I felt bright lights in my face. I sat up and there looking in our window smiling down on us were the next passengers waiting at the train stop. I closed the shades. Our next stop ice fishing. Did I say I hate the cold? I literally had to buy a Canadian coat it was so cold.

I love my excursions with both Lily and Henry. Like their genre of movies, our trips together were the ying and the yang. Like the romance and action movies - I love them both

Continue making memories with your loved ones, even if it's camping in your backyard. Laugh your life away. In the end, it's your imagination. It's your journey. And it's still your day—until it's not. I always wanted to get the last laugh. Oh, make sure they keep your red cape.

Hug Always

Lie in bed with your partner. No words, just fierce hugs and perhaps tears. COVID took away those friend hugs that I dearly loved but my family knows the importance of keeping me safe with their warm embrace. We still get together, but always first get a COVID test if we are going to be staying together. This also allowed us to give big hugs. Life feels so normal when you can hug your family. We are all vaccinated, but still you can never be too safe especially when you have Stage IV cancer.

Tired of quarantine, my immediate family and I decided to escape Nashville and go on a secluded beach trip to an island near Charleston. We drove of course. We secured a great house on the beach at a great price because everyone was staying home. Everything was closed except a seafood and a meat market and of course one grocery store. We went to the beach every day, cooked every meal, played tennis (we were are all so bad) on empty courts, rode bikes on deserted bike paths, played games, and watched shows my daughter suggested by way of Sony. Every evening, we sat on our amazing deck and talked and laughed about anything and everything. It got really interesting to listen to the stories of those who drank Ben's margaritas. At the end of the evening, we hugged—a little wobbly perhaps.

Physical touch is so important in life. Not only with humans, but with all living things. We have two French bulldogs and it's amazing when you give thought to these creatures' behavior. They are always happy and freely give kisses and hugs all the time. Our French bulldog, King Louie, was appropriately named. He hogs the bed, is always in the middle of my nap, and cries when he wants something. The other one, Paris, is very French, mostly aloof, but when love is needed, she'll come find you. Don't have an animal? Visit the zoo or volunteer at the shelter to walk animals. If they bite, bite them back and hug them and keep walking. You never know their prior journey. Remember we really can't walk in someone else's shoes but we can have empathy and even share our red cape in the moment.

When Lily and Henry were younger and would get mad at each other, I would sit them down next to each other. Then I would make them face each other and make them hug. This often turned into laughter. See what happens with a simple hug. Maybe if all the angry people these days should sit in a room and hug, it might be the start of solving the world's problems. If you need a hug and no one is around at the moment, grab that red cape and embrace its warmth.

Weed Out Friends

A friend is not the person whom you call crying and they respond "I'll come by" and 20 minutes later call you to say it's too late and not show up knowing that you are alone and having a dark day. Yes, this happened to me. Wake up. If something like this happens to you or has happened to you, please know that a friend would not leave you hanging. This is an acquaintance and falls off the friend list. Your BFF will come over to cry with you to laugh with you and to pick up your red cape, snuggle with you in it for the moment, and remind you that you are a superhero.

What's really important is whom will you ask to be there for you when you come home from the hospital with tubes sticking out everywhere and knowing you have no breasts. It's shocking to see. Don't ever ask a mastectomy person if you can look. Ever. I think I pretended it wasn't me. I had to survive this mental overload. Those tubes had to be milked and I had to take tons of medications and then there is the recovery.

I chose Nadine to come stay with me after my surgery. She is a great friend and a nurse practitioner, which was a Godsend, but I chose her because of her spirit and laughter. We got home from my long day of surgery and of course I am on more drugs than Walgreens keeps on their shelves. Nadine promptly sat me and Ben down at our kitchen table, pulled out an expensive bottle of red wine with three glasses. Even drugged, I'm thinking why a third glass. She said, "We're all drinking and celebrating your recovery and your road to remission." And we did. I can't remember the last drop, but I can promise you I laughed and slept like a baby on that horrible mentally painful day, thanks to Nadine. She stayed two weeks and by day three we were shopping at the mall with my tubes tucked inside a belt I had bought on the internet. I had visitors that showed up and said where is Liz? Ben said oh, she's shopping. Imagine their faces.

My recovery was remarkable, and I owe it to my home caregivers:

Ben and my happy-go-lucky nurse and best friend, Nadine. Laughter is medicine and healing. Those two weeks that red cape took a break (except for naps) - but it was always a chair away.

I have so many friends but honestly I have only a handful that I know I could call right now and they would drop everything if needed. I am at peace knowing who they are and knowing there are other acquaintances in my life that play a role.

I have a very negative family member (related by marriage) that was toxic to the very end until I finally cut her off. She brought about such negative energy that I would be angry for days. Literally at my brother's death bed, she told me, "Your brother's doctor said he would die in five years from his metastasized bone cancer, and yes, Liz…today is right around five years. I guess you have two years left before you die." If I hadn't been so in shock over my brother dying, I would have knocked her out.

Maybe I will, maybe I won't die in two years, but I'm not going to let anyone dictate to me my outcome. Can you even imagine? My wonderful holistic therapist told me to walk out of these relationships forever because I was in the fight of my life and I didn't need these types of fights. I just deleted, or as they say these days, I "canceled" her by deleting her from anything where we were attached. It was cathartic. Today, only supportive, fun friends, who are helping my journey.

If you need to re-assess your true friends, grab that red cape and go down memory lane. Tie their name to a balloon and let it go.

Chase Marco Polo

Download the Marco Polo app, and create groups (family, friends, etc.). It is such a delight throughout the day to see snippets of live videos that will make you smile, laugh and want to participate. Both my family and Ben's family started Marco Polo and for such a long time it was the most fun. It slacked off after things opened back up and we all became busy again. But I still use it from time to time and I still see the value.

I remember how we would all laugh at my sister. No matter who posted, she would literally repeat the post and then say something nice. It drove us all crazy. (My sister only knows this by reading this now. Ha!) To make these moments even more entertaining, my sister's husband would initially post videos where we would only see inside his nose. Angles are important, people. Family can be brutal when you make a mistake, but that's what makes things funnier.

Ben's sister used to whisper in her videos and we weren't sure why but her brothers loved to pick on her. They would post a Marco Polo mimicking her with their own story. I'm telling you there were laughs every day. Thank goodness we all have lizard skins and can laugh at ourselves. With tons of love flowing to every home, the Marco Polo videos were the highlight of my day. It's cool how the chase of technology can help you find your smile.

No makeup. No groomed beard. No problem. Just press the fun buttons to change your face, your voice and remember to adjust your red cape. The point is to show up because it's no fun not being a part of the fun. Thanks, Kathy for sharing this app.

I encourage you to try this app or find your own app that brings you laughter and keeps you in touch with loved ones.

PART V: Exercise for Your Health

There are many stress relievers, I guess. But simple exercise not only heals the soul but works that lymphatic system. It creates flow and removes toxins from the body. Don't think one and done. Exercise is not running or walking three miles and then sitting afterward for the rest of the day. This negates your work. You must persevere. Look at that red cape, fold it up, and grab that red bandana and maybe those red shorts for now and go! Just start somewhere. Just start. Think 5 minutes every hour. One way you can find fun exercise is by buying a mini trampoline and jumping 10 minutes a day (or longer or shorter virtually). It's therapeutic and it is one of the best ways to get your lymphatic system moving. Don't forget to lift a few weights two or three days a week. Think one exercise for each body part: large muscles and then small muscles: chest, biceps, legs, glutes, back, triceps, and abs. Then do two sets with high reps if using a very light weight or 10-12 reps with heavier weights times three sets. Find the time to exercise for your health and to increase your longevity.

Move Often

Don't you dare feel sorry for yourself now that you've been diagnosed (after you scream, of course). Get up and walk every day. Perhaps you only feel like walking to the mailbox, do it! Do something. All steps are not created equal when you have cancer, but with that red cape you can do anything. Buy newly released Radical Hope, 10 Key Healing Factors from Exceptional Survivors of Cancer & Other Diseases, by Dr. Turner and Tracy White. This book follows the *Radical Remission* book with a new #10 factor: exercise. This doctor admits it should have been in the first book. It has always been in my book.

In my 60s, I still move, but I move differently. No more marathons, now I hike or walk. No more road biking, now I e-bike. No more giant tennis courts, now I now play pickle ball. No more lifting weights for an hour. Now I lift for 30 minutes. Now I love my mini-trampoline. Best of all, most of these activities I do with friends.

In Nashville, we are blessed with a 3100-plus acre park I am fortunate that it is only a 20-minute drive from my home. I have three different friends that I try to meet every week to walk. One of them is my 75-year-old friend Dan. He taught me these trails and roads over 20 years ago, and he still knows them better than anyone I know. He should do commercials for Nike. We also loved to bike together.

Funny story here with Dan. He and I would invite different people to bike with us. I'm talking bicycle. These friends were always from our gym where we were all so social. Honestly this is where I made my kind of friends because they all loved doing the same things as me.

One day, Dan's friend showed up to ride bikes with us dressed in full motorcycle gear. We snickered as they say, and went on the ride—a road bike ride that is—the one with the skinny tires and 27 gears. About 20 miles in, at the top of the last very steep hill, he literally fell over and said curse words even I had never heard. Sweaty, red faced from heat and madness, his friend swore he'd stick to motorcycles from that day on. And he did. The others and I, however, kept riding our bicycles while laughing many days about this story.

It has been over 20 years and my friend Dan is a testament to exercising. He taught high school and coached football, he ran short races, biked tons of miles, swam like a fish and still does these things with modifications. He walks now and bikes shorter distances, but he still swims like a fish. He has inherited health issues that he still deals with but by golly it doesn't stop him. And this is how I am living my life. Cancer is something I am living with, but it is not dominating my day.

My other exercise friend is Judy. Did I mention that after having been friends with her through my divorce, those running days became therapy for me. She is the friend who introduced me to Ben. We were scheduled to go on a blind (double) date with her and Seth, her husband. They both claimed they had the stomach flu. I figured Ben was safe as they knew him for years, so I still went on the date.

Now I was living in a small house with a tiny front yard. It was the Christmas season and I had one of these spiral trees outside that someone had stolen, and I had to buy another one. This time I nailed it down and tied it to my big tree with the fake owl, which was obvious up close. Ben arrived, saw this, laughed and said I fell in love when you opened the front door and I saw your face and your barking little dog.

I was an obnoxious back seat driver and all the way to the restaurant, I kept thinking he was going the long way. It's a continuing funny story in our family when anyone rides with us to this day, I still tell Ben which way to go and basically how to drive. Any who, we closed down the restaurant and four months later we were secretly married. When you know you know. Thank you, Judy. Yes, Judy is still marathoning, but she is kind enough to take it easy and walk with me. She's my amazing triathlon friend that is bored now because she is the only one in her age group at most races at age 68.

Judy also introduced me to my friend Susan through biking. We biked 40-plus miles two days a week. Most of the time three ladies never work well together, but we called ourselves "the three amigos." About 15 years later, we realized we should have been called "the three amigas." I never did learn Spanish. ☺ Not only did we bike for years, but we also traveled together. You learn a lot about friends when you travel with each other. Judy lightly snored, Susan screams at people in her sleep, locks herself out of her room, forgets her safe code in her room, and always has to have her own room that is sometimes connected to ours. She still makes us laugh today. We are all still great friends and still travel together just less often.

My friend Jan and I go back the farthest. She's very busy now so we don't see each other often, but we talk every week. Honestly, she grew up with me through moving to a new city, running our first marathon, and both going through a divorce at the same time, which was the cause of our first marathon. To this day I can confess anything to her and know she understands. She says when she feels like crap, she thinks about me and what my daily struggle must feel like and slaps herself as a reminder that she is the lucky one. I agree, cancer sucks, and it can eat at you minute by minute but your mind-body connection is stronger than your cancer. But thanks Jan for remembering there is always someone struggling worse than us. Be kind when you haven't walked in another's shoes or sat through the horrifying news that you have cancer.

My friend Boo started out shuffling her feet when we used to run, but now she can outpace walking most other people's running pace. She can talk the whole time to boot. She pushes me but only to the point she knows is not hurting me. Again, a friend for over 20 years.

My friend Ben—yes my awesome current husband of almost 20 years—is another exercise partner. Many of our dates each week consisting of him running with me on my many routes. In fact, the day after we got secretly married, we ran the Nashville half-marathon. I whispered to Judy at the start line that we had gotten married by the Justice of the Peace.

We had another family wedding three months later. We both had young children and didn't want to live together in front of them so we eloped and only our children and parents knew about out marriage. Funny story about our "fake" wedding (we knew no one would come if they thought we were already married), one of my clients, a Judge, married us. He kept asking me days before, "Liz, where is your marriage license," I said, "Don't worry, I'll get it." He married us thinking we didn't have it. I never did tell him. For 18 years even we were confused and celebrated our anniversary on the wrong day. It was only when we moved recently and found our marriage certificate that we realized our mistake. What the hell, a gift is a gift. Ha!

Travel was another way for Ben and me to get in our exercise. It was important in planning our trips. For example, one of my favorite trips to date was a European river boat cruise that we did a few years ago. We were by far the youngest couple on board, and the only Americans. When the boat would dock every day (for the entire day usually until early the next morning), we would literally run to get off first. Otherwise, you'd be waiting an hour behind the "old" people. Once off, we would explore the immediate town. All of these explorations were on our own. Then we would venture off. One example of how brave we were was renting an electric bike, which we'd never done. You can get as much or as little exercise on one of these bikes I discovered. The man handed us an old-fashioned map of the wine country which was somewhere in remote Germany. We didn't look at our watches it was so freeing and fun - until we needed to look at our watches. We did get lost. Perhaps the wine influenced our way. Lucky for us it was a midnight departure.

Part of this trip was a train ride after the boat ride to the Matterhorn. Of course it was snowing so we ditched this part of the trip and took off on our own to Switzerland. Ben and I are both spontaneous in our adventures and that is one of the things that makes us soulmates.

I love my time with these friends in Nashville and look forward to every activity whether it be walking, shopping (we get lots of steps), or having a nice conversation with a glass of my sugar free red wine. Being social with positive people is one of the best medicines you can add to your journey. It's healing and a way to boost your happiness. And when you boost your happiness, you're more inclined to want to move more often. So, my advice is to move. Instead of breakfast in bed, walk to grab breakfast and walk home. When you return, if you are tired, grab that red cape and take a nap. A nap after a walk is a well-deserved nap.

Embrace Your New Normal

Your blood work, your energy, your attitude, may all be on a roller coaster. Remember, you will find your new normal. Don't compare yourself, just treat yourself to small victories.

My brother who also had cancer, would call me on his lab day and we would compare our labs. Secretly, mine were always better, but I would always say, "That's great, you're doing so well," or "You need to take more supplements," or "Why aren't you walking or lifting weights?" I talked him into a trampoline and a treadle so he could do something inside to avoid the heat and cold. My friend, once you buy exercise equipment, you should use it at least. Encourage the person you know to find their new normal by finding something that works for them currently, like buying a mini-trampoline or bike of any kind, walking, hiking, or going to the gym. As for me, one of my new normals was stopping my marathons and starting to walk.

As an Exercise Physiologist by background, I have always exercised in some fashion and perhaps my undiagnosed attention deficit disorder also encouraged this movement. In September 2021, in JAMA, an article was published that talks about steps. You may have heard 10,000 steps is the magic number. After studying over 2,000 participants for over 11 years, ages 38 to 50, taking into account body mass index, smoking and other factors that could have affected findings, it was discovered that the magical number is actually 7,000 to 10,000 steps per day. Any steps beyond the 10,000 did not show any added benefit to health. But this 7,000 to 10,000 showed the greatest reduction in mortality risk. These steps do not have to be taken all at one time. It's amazing how many steps you get in by cleaning the house, walking your dog, or taking a short walk after your dinner.

There are going to be days when you may not make that number, but it is important to start walking as part of your cancer routine. My doctor always says to me, "Liz, are you still walking," and I respond,

"Yes ma'am. I walk every single day." She always says, "Don't stop." So, like my doctors ask me, my question to you is, do you make an attempt to walk every day? If not, I encourage you to make walking a part of your daily routine and over time, you will build up your endurance. Even if it is to your mailbox and back, walk. Remember not all steps are created equal when you are dealing with cancer.

Take note of where you are in your chemo cycle, I try to schedule my scans and labs the week I am rebounding from chemo. Often this hasn't been the case and I can tell a difference in my labs. Listen to your body when it is tired, knowing that this new normal may mean you have to take a longer nap on some days or weeks to refresh your mind, body and soul. But try to get in that walk. Wash that red cape on your good day. It will get smelly after exercising.

Download Helpful Apps

I just can't end this chapter as an Exercise Physiologist without offering some exercise advice. When I am traveling, I see people doing an exercise wrong and in my best southern manner, I correct their form.

Often people are happy, those that aren't will think about me later when they get an injury. One of those people happened to be Reba McEntire. I was in Florida on vacation working out in this tiny gym. We were the only two there at the moment. After I gently corrected her, she asked to work out with me. It was an aha moment, and she loved that I was from Nashville. Yes, I did train some country music greats but honestly I'd rather train my grandmother as she puts a lot less pressure on me and actually listens.

Sometimes when I travel, I pick five body exercises and do them in three rounds - three sets is the proper term. My poor travel mates are expected to join me. On my last little family trip, my cousin asked my sister, "Does Elizabeth still exercise?" and my sister responded, "Of course." They both started laughing knowing what was in store for them.

Exercising changes as we age. Age makes us slow down even if we still feel like a super star. I loved my running years and even now when I'm sitting on my front porch in Nashville and see groups going by, I reminisce. I ran marathons to get those lovely medals but mostly for the camaraderie of the training that takes place the many months before. We talked about everything, cursed at our pain, laughed at anyone who dared used a port-a potty instead of the woods. Real runners don't use port-a potties. Ever! When I ran the NYC marathon, there was a sign that read: **Anyone caught peeing outside of a port-a potty would be kicked out of the race.** Whoa! I was scared, until I saw so many guys peeing off the first bridge we crossed. I had to laugh. Now I could run knowing the real rules: the runner's rules.

I started a training group at my husband's company to run a half marathon. What a fun way for employees to get to know each other and to see the real CEO and his crazy wife (that would be me). These conversations veered into talks of tag-team runs called The Ragnar Relay. Each team had 12 runners who would run a total of 200 miles non-stop. We had two vans of six. Six stinky sweaty people all in one van—sleeping, laughing, changing clothes, and jumping out of a Van at three in the morning. I, of course, gave everyone their duties. It was easy. Srini was to bring a few garbage bags in case someone needed it for the rain. I took peanut butter sandwiches—two bags worth—to keep us going until we could have a real meal. The others brought towels for our van and Reggie gave out the three-leg distances to each member of our team. Did I say they were all different distances!!

The reality: I was the next runner to run in the pouring rain. I looked at Srini who handed me a bag - a small trashcan bag that wouldn't even fit over my head. Reggie handed out our three legs and who do you think got the most miles? Me. The marathoner. I jumped back in the van soaking wet and went to grab MY towel but oh, it had already been used and was already wet. Did I mention that mine was a real towel and not a hand towel that the guys brought. That sandwich I couldn't wait to eat, well, Srini had devoured both loaves in their entirety. Even through all this lack of sleep, a smelly van and tired legs, it was the most fun. I know I must be crazy as I did this more than once. But I got Reggie back by dragging him to Berlin to run the Berlin marathon. It takes a little bit of crazy to be this type of runner. Crazy I love.

Now I walk. When I go out walking every morning, I turn on my Runkeeper app. You choose, running, walking, biking, and skating - just about any activity you can think of. This is a great way to take a new direction every day. I have mine set to say out loud "mile 1" so I can judge my distance. I can mindlessly walk, call a friend or listen to a fun book on audible. Not to mention, my Bose sunglasses are the bomb. They have a built-in microphone on the rim so I don't have anything stuck in my ears. Honestly, I sweat out those ear pods that everyone loves. They were my gift to me for exercising outdoors. You can buy them online. They make great Christmas gifts too.

On the days that I strength train which for me means lifting weights or lifting kettlebells, I walk a shorter distance either before or after my workout, But for my weight training, I warm up on my mini trampoline. It not only is a great warmup for five minutes but it works the lymphatic system. Nassau just did a study that showed that the mini trampoline is the number one activity to reverse or prevent cancer. Ten minutes every day. I will do side-to-side steps, never jumping actually, then half-jumping jacks, twisting with my feet always touching, and finally high knees. I set a ten-minute timer and count about 25 for each one then repeat. You can start just with steps and fewer minutes. I don't use the bar that comes with it, but if you are not well-balanced, it is a good idea to put it on. You can always take it off later. The amazing thing about this mini trampoline is I also use it to do some of my weight training since I don't have a leg machine anymore. I put a weight or kettlebell in both hands and step up with only one foot on the trampoline. Using only that one foot, I stand straight up and add a shoulder press with the opposite arm. It's a great strength builder for the legs and shoulders. You can also do pushups and sit on it to work your abs or to just rest.

Having fitness trained for over 20 years, I learned so much. At age 50, I went back to college to get my Masters in Exercise Science, and I obtained so many fitness certifications that I was classified as a Master Trainer (nationally certified). I never asked a client to do what I had not done. When you seek a trainer, it is important to ask about their fitness background and their fitness education. Don't get injured with an unqualified trainer.

Before you start to strength train on your own, download the Tabata Pro app. It allows you to plug in the number of exercises, your warmup time between sets, your number of sets (tabatas), and your rest time in-between your exercises. It makes you work harder and smarter. I have always used this wonderful app. It allows you to work without focusing on counting. I suggest starting with seven to eight exercises for 30 seconds of work, 15-20 seconds of rest, and two sets. A warmup of three minutes to five at the most. This is if you are a beginner. If you are not a beginner and have been working out, I suggest 8-10 exercises for 40-45 seconds of work, a 10 second rest, two to three sets (only two if you are 60 or older), and your top number for starting should be 30 seconds and will be your rest between tabatas/sets. Do your warmup outside of the Tabatta Pro app. At least this is free advice to help you start an organized workout.

One of my favorite weights today is the kettlebell. It really is the biggest bang for your buck when you are strength training. Every time you lift a kettlebell you are working your abs because the weight is not equally balanced like a dumbbell. You can buy them at target, online, or at Dick's Sporting Goods. I always have clients start with a 5lb, 10lb, 12lb, and 15lb if they are a woman, and for men a 10lb, 15lb, and 25lb. You can find workouts online. I strongly suggest working out in front of a mirror to make sure your form is correct or better yet, have a few sessions with a nationally certified trainer (not one that got a certificate online or had a one day session). If something hurts when you are working out, you probably have bad form.

Most importantly, cancer changes your energy at the end of your chemo. That would be day 15 for me as I take a pill 21 days straight (then off seven days), or a week after your liquid chemo. Always listen to your body, but let your mind find a way to do something even for 10 minutes. After you are done, pat yourself on the back, grab your red cape, and rest.

PART VI: Discern Mind Games

Focus on you all the way to radical remission. Ponder writing a funny story, a life story, and/or an inspirational story. The point is when you let your mind play games, your body follows suit. Shut it down, my friend. Your mind game is your healing, your kick-ass healing.

How are you?

How am I? Well, how the hell are you? I'm so tired of this question when it's referring to me being sick. Do I look sick? Do I have the letter C written on my forehead? Am I being a complainer? Shut the F up and just be yourself with me. I'll let you know when I need sympathy. I promise I will be the first to speak up for help. And you better let them know you need help.

I have my breakdown moments, honestly I do. The tears flow like Niagara Falls - mostly with Ben. He knows to hug me fiercely and maybe cry with me. It is important to let it out. To me, holding back tears is like holding your breath. The longer you hold your breath, the more you can't breathe until you are blue in the face or faint. I don't look good with a blue face, so I'll cry. Let those damn tears and frustrations flow like a river but only for a short time. Maybe not share this with the person that always asks "how are you" unless you want awkward stares and/or unwanted advice.

My mother, bless her soul, was a constant complainer about her health. I would try to warn everyone that called her or visited her, do not ask "how are you" because you would listen for the next hour to every ailment that is humanly possible both real and imagined. It never failed that Ben would forget and I would be laughing on the sofa as he tried to move this conversation to another topic. You probably know someone like this too. Funny thing, my mother will outlive us all.

When people know your diagnosis, they do treat you differently and I guess some people like that attention, I don't. I want to be treated like a human not a cancer victim. Cancer wins when you give in, cancer wins when it consumes how you are. Kick it to the curb. My Utah friends never ask me this question because I chose to only reveal my cancer to a few friends out there and explained that I was as healthy as them in so many ways, and I wanted to be treated like a non-sick person. They may text me and ask how is Nashville treating you and tell me that they miss me, but they never ask "how are you?" Smile.

Again, I do have my days where I want to curl up and cry, but I grab that red cape because there are no tear stains on that, I get up, and my mind tells me to get up and go because this journey is not over. I have way too many reasons to live. *How am I?* I am fucking great.

He/She is Better Off

Oh she is better off now that she has died. Really! How the hell do you know? Don't look at me when I die and say this as you will promptly be removed from my exceptionally fun memorial service (planned by me). I'm thinking everyone will be so upset that I may get cheated and I figure you have only a few "you" times: your birth, when you find your soul mate, your child's birth, and your death or passing as I really believe in Heaven. When it's my time that will be between God and me.

Being from the South, I don't think I've ever been to funeral that I didn't hear these words "he/she is better off." Two deaths that affected me the most in my life were my Dad and my brother, Michael (more commonly referred to as Mike). Both were sick when they died. My Dad had smoked for so long (never around us) and drank for so long (never saw him drink but saw him lit every time). He finally quit it all but became so mean and short with everyone that I wanted to slip him a bottle of vodka. Too bad then I didn't know about pot gummies.

For almost 10 years he lived on oxygen and it was so sad to watch. In his final days, the oxygen literally left his body. At his funeral, he had lost so much weight that his glasses made him look like Mr. McGoo. In case you are not from the South, the casket is left open for everyone to walk by and say, "He/She is better off." My dad's was the first and only dead body I touched. I realized he wasn't even there at the moment. I looked up knowing that he was smiling as I was uneasy looking at those giant glasses on his face. I smiled back.

My children were very young and totally freaking out over seeing their Poppy dead. I didn't quite realize the trauma, the nightmares, and the questions. Especially the one on why Poppy was better off.

Funny story here, Ben and my ex rode from Nashville together to the funeral. Being that my mom always loved my ex more than me,

73

he was not only invited to my dad's service, but he was a pall bearer. I can't imagine the stories in that car but when you have confidence, you just shake it off. We are all still friends.

What I realized at his funeral was how everyone came together, like 9/11, and how everyone laughed and told their stories about my Dad. It was his day but one of my saddest days. He always, always listened to my stories, he listened to my made-up songs on my tiny organ/piano, even when he was lit.

The death that affected me the most, however, was my brother, Mike, the one who died of cancer. I remember when his cancer metastasized to his bones. His wife called my sister and me to come with them to Florida as it could be his last trip. He would probably die really soon. At the time, my cancer was having a happy dance in my body which I was unaware. My sister and her husband (my real brother to me), rushed to Florida trying to find a place at the last minute. I remember being scared for him to go in the ocean, walk very far or even ride a bike, thinking it would his last day that day.

Fast forward, five years later, Ben was driving 100 mph to get me to the hospital to say my last goodbye to my brother. He had already lost his voice. I cried the entire five hours. It was the middle of COVID and luckily he was at a little Catholic hospital close to his lake house. That hospital wasn't a COVID hotspot as they were sending these patients to another hospital, but all around Georgia was COVID. Vaccines weren't yet available. They were kind enough to allow us into his room—all 15 of us. Did I say we come from a huge family? My mom was one of 12 siblings and my dad one of 9 siblings. I had so many first cousins on both sides I never knew loneliness. I might add here when I looked around the room only a few of those people had on the required masks. It's a small town filled with stubborn "they don't tell us what to do" people.

Having Stage IV cancer, I was initially scared, but Mike was more important at that moment. When I saw him, my world stopped. My first thought was to tell him why he was so important in my life. We literally talked every day sometimes about cancer, and sometimes just about life. I would just listen to him go on a tirade about politics, a family member, or the fact that my daughter lived in California which made him crazy. At his death bed, he squeezed my hand so I knew he was listening. I saw the tears in his eyes, and he saw mine. I hated I couldn't hear his voice. I still sit today, close my eyes and listen for his voice. Tears come first every time but then a big smile.

After talking to him, I backed away for others but as I looked around that room, I knew my brother would not be happy that everyone was staring at him just waiting for him to die. I left. I was so angry at his doctor for giving him a statistic of five years, Even now, I can't let my mind go there because I'm close to four years with my metastasis and I still hear those words. Don't let anyone ever give you this type of statistic as it will mess with your mind. The mind-body connection is very real.

Mike had decided to be cremated on his death bed, which didn't surprise me because we both felt and feel the same about open caskets. I realized that Southerners find closure in seeing the dead body. I'm not sure why except maybe just seeing a dead body makes death real. That's another saying from Southerners, "I need closure" referring to open caskets. He hung on for days and he was in great pain. He lost his sight and I left before his last breath. This was my big brother, the one who was my rock when my parents were fighting, the one who made me laugh at dinner, the one who told me the real deal about Santa, the one who bailed me out when I got in real trouble (not telling my parents), and the one who shared my cancer diagnosis. We were connected and now, this connection was stolen away because of cancer. If I could kick cancer right now I would. Cancer fucking sucks!

When I first got the call in Nashville, I screamed. He had fought so hard, I was hoping for a miracle. I screamed thinking of my own cancer, thinking if I get sick, I want my nurse friend Nadine to bring that bottle of wine and overdose me on something quick.

I realized that people say these words, he/she is better off, because maybe they feel better off. No more care takers, no more worries, no more pain for them watching their loved one in their cancer journey. Their loss comes later. Okay, I get that, but don't you come to my memorial and say these words.

There will be no regrets either. What? No, no regrets - forgive now, love now, read more, travel more, move more, say you're sorry more, learn to say no to those energy suckers and get rid of those people that tell you when you will die. Regrets make us focus on stress, and as humans with a cancer diagnosis, we must focus on the glory of each morning, the blessings we have now, the gratefulness of life now, the joy of the quiet mind and listening to nature's sounds. This is our life now. This is your life now. Live in the now. This you will not regret.

I will be at the pearly gates with my red cape looking for my Dad and brother - and only then will I drop my cape for good.

So Many Worries

Don't let worry consume you. Instead, pretend every day that you are researching for the person you love the most. If you let this consume you in a depressed way, you will miss out on remission. You are the lead team member of this team you have created - consider yourself CEO.

There are days when I feel like I am in this battle alone. That is why it is important to find your cancer friends that think positively. Those who can share what they are researching or what they are doing that may be different from your daily routine. Ben still works and when I break down and cry and admit I feel alone in this battle, he stops and says let's look at this together, or let's have a conversation with other cancer centers or doctors. Sometimes you have to remind your loved ones that you need help.

Scans are always a huge worry - if you have cancer I know you feel me on this one. For me it's not the actual scan anymore, but the day wait in-between to see my doctor to receive the news. On this day, I admit I take a gummy infused with THC and CBD - called a calming gummy right before bed. I sleep like a baby and honestly, it's better than valium.

Nashville is slow to recognize this for terminal ill patients but where there is a will there is a way. I boldly bring my pot gummies in my carry-on bag home from Los Angeles. I take a black permanent marker and color in the words on the can "pot infused," along with the pot symbol. Think they are going to arrest a Stage IV cancer lady? Just in case I do get arrested, please help me get out of jail. Social media is fierce these days. ☺

Worry creates stress and stress can eat you alive. Try to wake up and live like you don't have cancer. Pretend your cancer is like someone living with diabetes. It's there, for now, but please don't let it stop you or take a day away from you.

Cancer is expensive. That can bring about more worry, but there is money for you. Research, find it, accept it from a friend, ask your doctor - don't let this stop your journey. It truly is not fair for people that can't afford to reach out beyond their western medicine doctor if they choose. Don't let this stop you. Don't ever be afraid to ask whomever you are calling if there are organizations that can help you. Believe, my friend, believe. Grab that red cape to relieve that stress and keep it on for now so you can be bold and find the help you need.

Remember what your mom told you, "Where there is a will, there is a way." I did listen to mom every once in a while.

PART VII: Write Your Story

Cancer today, but what does your tomorrow hold for you? As for me, I'm striving for radical remission. I'm striving to be stable to no cancer. In the course of this journey, however, I realized that whatever the outcome, I want to be the one to write my story. Cancer, or no cancer, everyone should write their own story all the way to the end.

Lingering Memories

Talk about memories to your children. Write them down. This is fun writing. Tell your story, even those down-and-dirty secrets you never told anyone. Just publish it A.D. (after death) if you did something really bad. There are so many stories you will forget to share or just forget until you start writing them down. The good, the bad, and the ugly of your experiences may inspire someone or maybe just make them smile on a bad day.

Writing this book over the past two and a half years has made me think about my life. I was a wild child looking for attention without knowing it. Being the youngest of four—two older brothers and one older sister—I learned to be street smart and home smart. How to blame someone else (I still do - ha ha), how to fend for myself because my mom and dad did not dole out money without a fight are a few of my character traits.

I worked at a movie theatre when I was 16. It was my first real job not working with my dad on his construction sites painting. My dad loved that I was working at the movies because I would bring home the leftover popcorn every day. We both loved popcorn. My friends expected free tickets but I was lean and mean and never gave one free ticket - made me a great sales manager later in life.

What was interesting about this first job of mine was the owner. He was a fat, dirty old man. I recognized that from day one and kept my distance. I needed this job and money to pay for my car insurance and clothes. My sister's friend worked there also (three years older than me). I saw him harassing her and I'm not sure if anything ever happened as this was a day and time that these things were hidden and you didn't ask. However, I remember thinking at 16, no man would ever take advantage of me like that. I would kick him in the balls and punch him in his Adam's apple if I ever felt threatened. This was the start of my many plots in my mind to overcome my fears. Maybe a little crazy but I never had to deal with bullshit harassment.

My fondest memories were in my 20's and 30's. I put myself through college, working full-time and going to night school full-time. Sometimes I found time to date but it never worked out that I had a boyfriend. I just never had the time to devote to anyone. I did my fair share of partying as this didn't require anything except aspirin the next morning.

I thought this was out of my system at my current age, until I hosted a pool party in Utah for all my new girlfriends - ages 45-65. You could hear the music across the desert, and we laughed and danced and drank until 1:00 in the morning. I will admit I let them keep drinking long after me. Don't worry we all live in the same neighborhood so no driving home, except a few golf carts weaving down the road. It's fun to feel free and crazy at times.

Back to my 20s, I always applied to jobs I wasn't qualified for but my confidence in my interviews always won me the job. I figured I was a fast learner so I could fake my way until I was actually good at the job. I knew I had to support myself in every single way. Landing a job at a prestigious Atlanta law firm helped pay for the rest of my college. It took me five years but I finished. I was the first in my family to obtain a four-year college degree. At 50, I went back to get my master's degree and this allowed me to finally be a teacher, which was my childhood dream. I taught at a community college and of all my career moves, this became my favorite job of all time. I was probably more mature than my counterparts in my 20's because I was a survivor, a street-smart young lady that thought she could do anything.

I didn't have a mentor so sometimes I would veer off course, like when I quit that great law firm job to move to Pensacola Beach with my girlfriend from high school. She didn't have to work, but as for me, I always needed a job. I interviewed with a criminal lawyer my first day there while my friend waited at a local bar to pick me up afterward. I stood on the side of the street waiting and waiting for her. There were no cell phones then, so I couldn't call. Finally the lawyer that interviewed me, drove by in his pink convertible Cadillac and offered me a ride home across that long bridge. It was a lengthy ride, but I got the job the next day. I realized very quickly that he represented all the bad guys.

It was an interesting, fun summer. My girlfriend left a few months later to teach in Germany at an air force base, and I stayed a while longer. I never regretted taking a chance. Luckily my old Atlanta boss hired me back eight months later. Funny, I never worried about money (or getting a job) even though no one ever gave me money. At the time, everything I owned fit in my Honda Civic. What a memory that I don't regret!

My 30s were powerful. This was the decade I had met my ex, who was a lawyer. Although we married when I was 32, we met when I was in my late 20s. Never did I dream I'd have children. I think I was consumed with being successful and afraid to be responsible for someone else. I landed the best job—once again way over my head—in telecommunications with what is now AT&T (but then it was BellSouth). I lived in Memphis, due to my ex's job, and discovered another world existed in this town. My ex and I were living together but planning on getting married. I always loved change, but this Atlanta girl was in shock going to Memphis. I learned to keep my southern mouth shut about cohabitation. We eloped and were married by an Indian Chief along a river in full cowboy lace hat and cowboy boots right after a beautiful hard rain. No one knew we had gotten married. It was magical. I called my mom the next day and she said she had a dream that I had gotten married. I guess mothers always know.

At age 35, I was expecting while living my best life, making a six-figure income managing a sales team. I was no longer a sales rep. This was before retail stores. Being a Sales Manager was stressful. It was challenging. It was highly competitive. There was never a day I didn't want to go to work. My counter-part Mickey and I would never let a day slide by that we didn't pick on each other. We were the top reps in the company in our region. I would announce over the intercom, "Mickey, your hairpiece has arrived." He would later announce, "Would my assistant, Liz, please come to my office." Our sales team loved it. Customer service loved it. Every month, we all, through humor, lifted our teams to number one and number two. (Mickey mostly was number two, ha! I get the last laugh here, buddy).

Once my sweet Lily was born, heck, I was almost 36. She was

now my purpose. For the first time since I was 15, I quit working, and I stayed home with her. Lucky for me, BellSouth missed me and I landed a once-a-month job traveling around the South teaching telephone operators how to bundle cellular with telephone sales while making the same amount of money and taking my family along. You know those pesky calls to up-sell, but in this case, people craved this service.

It was on one of these weekends, here in lovely Nashville, I discovered in a taxi, that I was pregnant with Henry at age 37. Living with no family in Memphis, I decided to stay home completely with both children. I never gave thought to our income sacrifice. I didn't care. I knew this was the right thing for me to do. I never regretted my decision.

This decision later led me to be a fitness trainer so I could manage my own days. Matt Royka (my friend and only fitness trainer) inspired me to become a fitness trainer. Did I say I think all the ladies hired him as he was Mr. Dreamy, but they had no idea they were getting the best kick-ass trainer on the market. We became fast friends. Seriously, I talked him in to starting a marathon training group so we could all suffer training together (even though he had not run a marathon) and 20 years later he's still training and hosting a marathon group. Being my "trainer hero," I decided he was right and I would pursue being a fitness trainer. This new career would fit my new life choice of working my own schedule so I could be a kind of stay at home mom. He never dreamed I would not only fitness train, but get my Masters.

At one point, I could do 10 full pull-ups. In fact, when I was making my national training video as part of my certification, I was in the gym with a friend who was videotaping me during the slowest part of the day for a gym. While demonstrating those same pull-ups for my test, I felt hands on my waist. Someone was assisting me with my pull-ups. All I thought about was how angry I was because I was being interrupted in the middle of my video. When I came down, I turned around and there stood the legendary country music star, Kenny Chesney. I asked him if he could help me get five more, and by the way, I kept the cameras rolling.

Confidence is powerful. Face cancer head on with the

confidence that you'll survive and thrive. Leave those life memories behind for your children, your family, or your friends to share. We focus so much on our careers, our children, and our relationships that we forget how we got to where we are—the good, the bad, the ugly. Memories help you deal with your present day, and the really good ones—that you can't discuss in this lifetime—can be read with wow and laughter when you are gone. Maybe in the end, I'll frame my red cape for them so they never forget.

Daily Gratefulness

Express your gratitude daily. Yes, your gratitude. Do it out loud if you can. You could be homeless, paralyzed, or even blind. You have a lot for which to be forever grateful. Here's a secret, expressing your gratitude will make you feel amazing on a daily basis.

Health and Science was one of the college courses I taught. This included topics like STDs, pot smoking, sex, and a number of other fun things for a professor to teach. It was awkward, but I decided if I had confidence in the subject matter so would my class. Knowing these were going to be uncomfortable topics, I decided to start the class with a few interesting introductory exercises.

The first day of class was an unusual introduction of 28 very diverse college students. This is why I loved teaching at Nashville State Community College. I split them in half and told them they had one minute to line up in order of how many siblings they had, largest to smallest, without talking. Not a word. It was a fun simple exercise that did three things: it got the students out of their comfort zone, it made them realize that body language is just as important as spoken words, and most importantly, it encouraged the students to work together and be grateful for their teammate.

The next day, we did a balloon exercise. Each person wrote one regret on a sticky tag, and if they needed more than one sticky, it was given. I had 35 balloons blown up the day before, at my expense, and each person placed their regrets around the balloon string. We stood in the courtyard of the campus and all said at the same time, "We are moving on and letting these regrets go with the wind." We let the balloons go at the same time. It was cathartic. I told the class, from that point on, we would be grateful, not regretful.

I loved this class, and I loved teaching. When I got the job offer I was so excited because I told Ben, not only was it a dream to teach when I was a child, but now people would really have to listen to me and do what I say. I was the youngest of four children so this was a big deal to me.

Back to the class.

My students voted me best professor after my first semester and said that I needed a raise so I wouldn't leave. Any great teacher— who loves their job—knows you don't teach for the money. The greatest benefit about adjunct professorship was that I didn't have to attend teacher's meetings or other faculty events unless I wanted. My wonderful dean, Julie, made sure I was one credit short of being full-time. I did not want to spend my days, weekends, and evenings in boring staff meetings and other tedious matters. She was, however, concerned when I stated that I gave out my cell phone number to my students. Honestly, this is the way young people communicate. Voicemail - they don't have a clue. So I told her it was no big deal because I told them if they texted me after 10:00 pm, I would text and/or call them at 5:00 am the next morning. It happened once. Word spread quickly, and it never happened again.

An important life lesson I wanted to teach my students was learning to be grateful so I had my class start a grateful journal for two weeks. Every single day they were expected to write down three things they were grateful. At the end of this two weeks, I stood up and selectively read what a student was grateful for that day from his/ her journal entry. We laughed, we were sad, and we were humbled. This was the last time I read as now they were a team, grateful for each other and not afraid, or mostly not afraid, to stand in front of their peers to speak. They spoke weekly. My goal was to prepare them for real life, real jobs, and real situations while reminding them to be grateful through it all. Out of this simple exercise, you awaken a peace and a love inside that makes you ready to go forward in your day. Although I'm not in the classroom anymore, I still abide by said gratitude principles. Early in the morning, I grab my red cape and remind myself of three things that I'm grateful. I encourage you to do the same.

Rejoice Today

Life…you only have it this one time: carpe diem. You are alive, rejoice! What do you do first thing in the morning?

Ben always arises first with our French bulldogs, and when I come down the stairs saying my "good morning, good morning" very loudly and happily, he hides somewhere and jumps out and scares me. It never fails. We both laugh and hug, and I sigh thinking, *Thank you God for giving me another day.* I don't take this for granted.

My mornings are basically the same. I guess this happens as we age. Wherever I am, I like to wake up early because, to me, the mornings are just the best time of day, next to sunset. After our little routine mentioned above, I grab my coffee, hug the dogs, and proceed to either write or read three different newspapers online. I also read my Bible verse for the day. (I like the Holy Bible app). On my morning walk, I say out loud why I am grateful. The rest of my day is unpredictable but my mornings are a reminder to me that I am alive another day.

An exception to these mornings is when I have my CT and bone scans. The night before, I pray that I continue healing as God promised according to the "ask and ye shall receive" Bible verse. I think God expects you to also work on your part of this equation. An outside-the-box example would be similar to the relationship parents have with their children. I have my kids' back no matter what, however, I expect them to work hard, to be kind to others, and to take care of their health through daily exercise and clean foods. They can ask me for anything, but I expect for them to do their part first.

Ask for help. Cancer does take a village, but before you ask for anything, when you wake up, your first thought should be to live today. Smother that cancer with that red cape while you have your coffee and imagine yourself healed. You, my friend, are ALIVE!

PART VIII: Personal Hygiene

I've always been a germaphobe, but it was heightened after I got the cancer news. I trained myself not to touch my face and to always, always have hand sanitizer. When COVID happened, I had stockpiles (even for my kids) thanks to my persistence with germs. My husband had the flu for three days before we knew it and I did not catch it and I'm sure it's because he immediately started wearing a mask when he knew he was sick. Any time there was a sick household member I had them mask up as well. This is Cancer, and even a small sickness has devastating effects on all of us. Wash that red cape often. Don't be embarrassed because you now have to demand no sick family or friends allowed over with that new cold or looming virus. Just say NO!

Masks are now acceptable, so wear them in public places even when none are required. Don't believe in them? Why did the flu practically go away when masks were required? Why did the common cold practically go away? Do what you must, but this is not political.

Looking good

Be diligent with washing your hands, and quit shaking hands. Think toilet hand. Gross! An elbow bump these days is totally acceptable. Take hot showers. They heal the soul as well as the aches and pains. It is important to look your best so you feel your best. My 98-year-old friend was very sick in the hospital but asked the nurse to get her red lipstick. Now that's the attitude. You're only as good as you look. Oh, wait. The expression is you're only as good as you feel, but my friend, I equate the two.

When I used to run those crazy marathons, my first thought when I got ready to run was do my clothes match? Do I look like a runner? Do I look like I can finish this race? Now at the end of the marathons, there was no way I looked good. I sweat like melting cheese in an oven. There wasn't a summer day running that I didn't wring out water from my socks and pour water out of my shoes. My running mates would stand amazed.

The night before a marathon, I would lay out my clothes, my shoes, and my socks in an orderly manner. I would wake up super early, have my coffee to make sure my system was working before running 26.2 miles. I would then take a shower, look in the mirror, and say to myself, *You can do this today, and oh, you look pretty good.*

I will admit one of my most embarrassing moments was in a 10K race in Nashville. Determined to win my age group, I refused to stop when I felt the urge to pee. When I crossed the finish line, there was a cute young guy taking the chip off the runners' shoes. I couldn't bend over because I was worried about developing a cramp from sweating. Guess what, the pee didn't stop. I literally peed all over the pour guy taking off that chip. I didn't have a water bottle with me, so he was very aware of what had happened. By the way, I won my age group. While I didn't look good at that moment accepting a trophy wet and stinky, I was full of confidence anyway. So maybe I did look good. Ha!

"Fancy" is Ben's favorite pet name for me. It always makes me smile. I love when he takes me on a date. No matter what I wear he always says "you look great fancy." He knows I love fashion whether it's exercising, running errands, or going on our date. If you don't think you look good, then throw on your red cape. It dresses up anything.

Remove Your Gross Shoes

Wear your shoes outside but not inside. Ditch them. Anyone who enters your home, make them also ditch their shoes. Fun fact: The oldest known shoe dates back to 3500 B.C. (before Christ). In Mesopotamia, soft shoes were introduced by mountain people on the border of Iran who ruled Babylonia during that time. They basically looked like moccasins. Shoes obviously progressed, but in these ancient times, it was customary to remove one's shoes before entering a home. In the Bible, God commanded Moses to remove his sandals before approaching him on Mt. Sinai.

Why am I sharing this? Because those diagnosed with cancer should be especially aware of all the germs lurking around them. There are reasons to remove your shoes. Let me explain why I think it is important. Those shoes have walked over a lot of gross, dirty surfaces, and you probably don't want that traction in your living quarters. Think about where you've traveled to throughout the day. Were you on an airplane in the restroom or in any public restroom? Think about what you've stepped over or on. Do you want to bring that into your home? If you don't think this is silly, take a swifter wet wipe and wipe that shoe on the bottom one day, or better yet, I dare you to lick that shoe if you think it's clean. Hmm. Exactly. *Gross!*

When I enter someone's home, I offer to take off my shoes. If they say no, I don't because I am worried about what is on their floors and what I will take home. You may think this is overkill. But imagine that I flew to Los Angeles from Nashville, or worse, drove. Think about all the public restrooms that I stepped in along the way. I read once that a public restroom has around two million bacteria per square inch. Knowingly, imagine I knock on your door and enter your home with those same shoes I just traveled in. *Eww.*

Studies have shown that 26% of shoes that are worn inside the home are contaminated with Clostridium difficile, a bacteria that can cause stomach pain and diarrhea. The University of Arizona researchers found that 96% of the bottom of your shoes also contain fecal bacteria.

Being immunocompromised with cancer, creates a higher possibility of infections from germs. Yes, something as mindless as dirty shoes can create infection for the immunocompromised. This, in and of itself, is the most important reason not to be embarrassed to ask guests, including family, to remove their shoes when entering your home.

I'm not saying you are going to die from shoes worn in your home, but why would you even think to allow bacteria in your sacred space that is unavoidable. Plus I'm my own housekeeper and it makes cleaning house a whole lot easier when there are no dirt from shoes. Even my pets get their paws wiped after going outside,

Please don't clean those shoes with your red cape.

Don't Stop Traveling

Traveling can be scary with cancer, especially when you are traveling by plane. Let's face it, it's a germ party in the airports as well as the planes themselves. Use wet wipes to wipe down the overhead bin, seatbelt, seat tray, arm rests, and screen buttons. Then use your hand sanitizer as often as possible. Avoid washing your hands in that bathroom. Instead use your hand sanitizer. Wear a mask. It becomes a habit.

You should not be afraid to travel, just be cautious. Nasty flight attendant? Now is the time to use the C-card just to make her feel bad. Don't be afraid to "fly." Even before COVID-19, I was doing all of these things. People looked at me like I was a freak. Now, everyone has to wear a mask, albeit I see many chin diapers—masks that are not worn to cover your nose. Nevertheless, don't hesitate to remind a seat mate to pull up their mask. "I have cancer." They are never ugly when you use these three words.

These days, when I wipe down my area after being seated, my seat mate often asks could they borrow a wipe. While we're talking about proper hygiene and safety precautions, please don't wear a cloth mask, but instead a real N95 mask when flying. When that person behind you takes off their mask, at least you are the most protected. Ben has caught so many things on a plane from traveling without a mask and not being aware of the germs around him (before the pandemic). I'm sure one day masks will no longer be required on flights, but my cancer friend, please keep yours on when you fly. See the world. Don't be afraid, just be cautious.

~

Funny story about one of my pre-COVID flights. Knowing the airlines never cleaned properly between flights, I would wipe down my area and put the dirty cloth on the floor near the aisle. I'd sanitize and sit back to relax. The flight attendant—who was gloved—came by to pick up trash. Mind you she was taking trash from customers. She got to me and said, "Can you hand me that nasty cloth?" I looked at her and replied, "If you don't mind getting it since you have on gloves and are picking up trash." She gave me the nastiest look and said, "It's not my job to clean the plane," and I said, "It's not mine either. And oh, I'm paying your salary." Guess who picked up the dirty cloth?!

The point is, extreme cleanliness is your new normal no matter what the world is doing. After all, personal hygiene is…well, personal. Why don't you grab a red mask with that red cape, COVID-style.

PART IX: Think Outside the Box

Remember the saying "there is a time and place…" Well, there is no better time than now to think outside the box. The inside of the box (traditional medicine) is a given, and that, my friend, at Stage IV has not sent anyone into remission - an extension of life, but not remission. So now you need to add thinking outside the box to your healing journey. Remission is possible. It can and it has been done. Your red cape is a start. Now the rest of you needs to get on board.

Releasing Pain: CBD and THC

CBD and THC? Why not? There are only benefits to CBD and if you decide to add the THC, then sweet remission dreams, my friend. CBD and THC both have been shown to complement cancer treatments by helping with nausea and vomiting from chemo and helping with neuropathic pain, metastasis pain (like the THC and CBD cream I use on my back for my bone metastasis), and increasing an appetite for those too sickly to want to eat. Personally, I don't smoke anything, instead I use the pot infused gummies at night. Seriously, ease your pain and comfort you gain (you can quote me). NOTE: It doesn't interfere with chemo, people. In fact, there is scientific evidence that it enhances chemo. I'll let you research this one. It's like driving to a destination. If you aren't the one driving, you probably aren't paying attention to the directions.

When I use my CBD/THC cream on my back where my cancer has metastasized, I sleep like a baby. The research I suggested is everywhere. Just Google "cancer and CBD/THC benefits" and you will find a plethora of PubMed, peer-reviewed articles related to this subject. I recently was in California and walked into a very nice store that looked like a pharmacy. The knowledgeable lady told me about a gummy that relaxes you for a good night's sleep. She told me to take half. I tried one that night when I went to bed and slept soundly, and I did not wake up feeling high or lethargic. Having this available when I know I can't sleep is comforting.

Funny story, my son told me to quit selling drugs in Utah. I was playing pickle ball and one of my friends, Dru, told me about her hip pain and how she couldn't remember her last good night's sleep. I proceeded to tell her about my calming gummies and she asked to please try one. I gave her one the next day on the courts. To my son's point, I guess I was handing off drugs in very conservative Utah. Ha!

That evening, Dru texted me to ask whether she should she take half or the whole thing. (Keep in mind, I only take half.) Well, I was at a dinner so I missed her text. I felt bad the next morning and texted her to make sure she was doing okay since I did give her pot. She was giddy while telling me she was ready to take me on a first class trip to Europe as she couldn't remember sleeping so well. Dru is witty, funny and beautiful and a damn good pickle ball player. I told her I would just settle to be her pickle ball partner. It cost me another four gummies.

Why is this seen as so bad? Cancer is bad. CBD/THC is helping me to get much needed sleep to heal, to go to bed without worrying about scans, my family, dying, or just what the next day will bring. This is your journey and you should make it as comfortable as possible. Former President Trump issued the Compassionate Care Act, and it's worth checking this out. Type in your search line "Compassionate Care Act" with your state's name.

Tennessee, where I currently live, is illegal to possess any THC products. However, I asked my oncologist about this care act and she said they could give me a medical letter but I had to first go through the behavioral health department at Vanderbilt. There, they would put me on "medicines" to see if those would work for my issues first, before allowing my official letter. Really? Bullshit on this unnecessary torture. More medicines, more looking at me like there is something mentally wrong with me for even wanting to take something so simple and non-toxic. I informed my oncologist that I would just keep packing it in my carry-on from California. If I get stopped and put in jail, I asked her to bail me out. If you read about me, please come protest outside my cell for all cancer patients to have access to this simple plant.

~

We have a great massage lady we use once a month. It's important to pay attention to your lymphatic system. She uses CBD/THC oil on my back because she is aware of my metastasis. She's so good I have to remind her about the pressure. *Whoa, horsey!* But it's the most wonderful feeling for your body to get a massage. Tell your family to gift you with a massage instead of flowers or a restaurant certificate.

It's a gift that keeps on giving. This reminds me I need to book her.

Do your research and experiment to see what works best for your cancer needs. You may need only CBD, but then again, you may discover THC. Grab that red cape, and get some well-deserved rest with your CBD or CBD/THC.

What Goes Down the Hatch?

When I first decided to juice it was because I read a book called *Chris Beat Cancer* by Chris Wark. I always thought of juicing as complicated and only for hippies. What I learned from Chris were three easy juice recipes that I use all the time. When you start juicing, you are feeding your body a vast amount of nutrient-rich fruits and vegetables. Your body, especially your kidney and liver, will kick into overdrive to remove toxins and also start to build newer, healthier tissues. There are so many health benefits I learned, including how juicing[7] can affect cancer cells.

I will admit I've tried over-the-counter juices and what I find is they taste too good. My advice is to look at those ingredients. If orange is the first one, then you can bet there are more oranges than carrots. It's very easy and cheaper to make juices yourself. But when you're on the run or traveling, and juicing is inconvenient, just beware of the ingredients or chose a place that makes the drink in front of you so you can ask for the ingredients that you like. There are many great organic green juice powders and plant-based protein shakes out there, too. Do what works for you because you will then be consistent.

There is a lot of work to taking care of my cancer. Sometimes I feel like I'm taking care of a newborn baby that is totally dependent on me. Oh, I am totally dependent on me. Some days when I feel overwhelmed, I may take the morning off and use only a plant protein shake. It can be liberating and much needed to get back on that horse.

I don't know about you but I had a bad sugar habit. That means I ate more sugar than fruits or vegetables. Did you know it only takes three seconds for that sugar sensation to reach your brain? This is quicker than a cigarette smoke buzz.

---

7 https://www.ncbi.nlm.nih.gov/pmc/articles/PMC526387/
https://www.ncbi.nlm.nih.gov/pmc/articles/PMC526387/

After reading and researching, the one common denominator I kept seeing was that sugar feeds cancer. Not berries--those are your friend (in moderation). I'm talking about the added sugars (e.g., cakes, cookies, candy) that give cancer its energy. It took me three full days to give up sugar, but I was determined to stop. Sweets for me was like a diamond necklace but now, I'd rather have the diamond necklace (hint hint, Ben). Sometimes, I'll still have a cheat day, and I admit it makes me feel so guilty.

Give up sugar now. Hurry. Think of it as a virus. *Yikes!* I wish I could teach my red cape to juice and to take away my sugar attempts. Since I can't, I'll just continue to do my part while asking God for healing and listening to the voices of Lily and Henry scolding me for reaching for sugar.

Going Meatless

Overwhelming evidence can be found on the topic of going meatless, especially for estrogen-driven cancer, but also for other medical issues. I reference here the books, *Blue Zones* by Dan Buettner *and Undo It* by Dr. Dean Ornish and Annie Ornish, as well as the many other books by these two pioneers. They are life-changers.

I eliminated meats and dairy from my diet as I have an estrogen-driven cancer. I've learned to love unsweetened almond milk and nutritional yeast for my cheese fix. Do I ever cheat? I recently was at Seaside, Florida (on 30a) with my daughter, my sister, and my cousin for a long weekend. They have these cute airstream trailers in town that host a variety of food and juices (these are gross so I know the greens are really greens). But one particular airstream that I loved before cancer, sells the best roasted chicken sandwiches I've ever eaten. Mind you, I haven't eaten meat in a very long time. So without an ounce of guilt, I walked up to the window and ordered my chicken sandwich with the baked beans and potato salad. I went all out. I savored every bite. I felt like a kid at Christmas. My insides didn't like this several hours later, but it was worth it in the moment. So yes, I have cheat days.

Going meatless is not easy when you have been a meat eater

your entire life. Although as a child, my mom would get so angry at me for refusing to eat meat. When everyone had my Dad's weekly steak, I would only eat the sides. At their favorite fish restaurant, I would ask for chicken noodle soup and hushpuppies. The worst to my mom, was my request every day for a mayonnaise sandwich on bread - nothing else. If you are wondering, I was always a skinny kid. Remember way back then there were no cell phones or computers, so I was always out riding my bike, playing street games or running barefoot with my cousins at my grandfather's place in the country. We used the pecan trees that lined the driveway for our forts and the working railroad track to run to the dime store. Our grandfather always had a stick of gum in his pocket for us and would remind us not to go inside his barn. That barn held his liquor steel. As if we couldn't smell it.

My best childhood memories were at his home. All my cousins (to many too count) would be there alternating Sundays. While the adults played horseshoes, we would play in those pecan trees, or run through the neighbors farm - all barefoot on dirt roads. Fondly, I remember my brother Mike, pulling me out of the cow pond as a bull was chasing us across the field in our Sunday clothes (we were told to change but too excited to be outside). My other two siblings were way ahead. Needless to say, you can imagine my mother's face when she saw our clothes.

I need to also say here, as you can't imagine, that when my Dad and his brother's (all seven of them) would drink and really get into their horseshoe game, that guns would come out if they thought someone cheated or was a smart ass. At this point, the women would yell "get in a car - any car, as we are out of here." My sister and I jumped in my Uncle Marvin and Doris' car in the back seat. No seat belts. He was driving like a drunk - oh he was drunk. For some reason, they thought all of us going back to the hotel would simmer the anger. Well, on this particular trip, Doris was cursing at Marvin until he opened her door and tried to push her out while driving 80mph. We were screaming, the car was swerving, yet somehow we made it back to the hotel - with Doris. There were always stories like this every single alternating Sunday. Perhaps, this is where my crazy originated.

Back to meat…

His neighbors would always host a cookout. I almost fainted when I saw an actual pig in the ground. This scared me for life and added to my disgust for meat. I think I had nightmares over this pig. This grandfather also had free range chickens and turtles. I would chase the chickens until one day, a rooster jumped on my back and started pecking me. He had to be pulled off by my grandfather who got the best laugh that day. He later, in front of us killed a chicken and turtle for dinner. No thanks. Another nightmare. These were my best times as a child. My one regret today are our children growing up with so much technology that they cannot relate to this type of childhood.

My other grandfather, my mom's Dad, who lived in downtown Atlanta was so far ahead of his time. He had a five-acre garden behind his home. I learned at an early age to savor beets, okra, and fresh tomatoes. I found a love for vegetables of all kinds. I guess you could say he was an organic farmer. He lived to be in his late 90s. If he had escaped Alzheimer's I think he would have outlived his 90s. Maybe my dislike of meat and love of vegetables was an early sign from God that warned me against meat. But as a kid, I never thought beyond the moment; now that's an aha moment.

Fun fact, this grandfather while a master Gardner, did not like children running around his house or yard. We thought he was a mean man because he would not let us ever play outside. He wanted us to just sit in the back room and talk. We were kids and do you think we sat in that room? As soon as the adults were settled in the front of the house, we would play hide 'n go seek using freshly made beds and closets to hide. I'll never forget when the covers were pulled back to reveal my grandfather's face. He would tell my mom to spank me and my cousin Dan. Ha! No one could ever catch either of us.

Another fun story at this same grandfather's house in Atlanta was the day Dan and I decided to stand across the street and see who could throw a rock in front of passing cars without hitting them. Mind you the city was exploding in growth and his street had become very busy. We were around 10 years old. As you can imagine, my rock hit a car window, and the car slammed on its brakes. We ran as fast as we could back to the house. It was so obvious as it was right across the street. The stranger knocked on the door. Luckily no was harmed, except my cousin and myself.

~

My adult years I discovered I liked meat. I think I ate meat twice a day. In other words, we do tend to eat like we did as a child. Grilled chicken and potatoes is a lot easier at first than figuring out a vegetarian or vegan meal. It is possible and really becomes easy when you look for the right recipes. I like recipe books like the books I mentioned earlier, but I also like finding recipes online. *Blue Zones* now has a meal planner which is also awesome and even prepares your grocery list.

I must insert other recipes I have gleamed from my reading and kitchen trials: *The Vegan 8* by Brandi Doming, *The Lean* by Kathy Freston, *Eating Purely* by Elizabeth Stein, "***lovingitvegan.com***," and many others. I'm not all vegan, not all vegetarian. I call myself pescatarian as I eat fish and eggs once every week. I don't, however, eat dairy. I also try my creative side to "make it up" with ingredients that have become staples. Sometimes it's great and sometimes we have to get takeout.

Grab your red cape and get busy trying healthy recipes. There is always take out if it doesn't work out.

PART X: Inside the Soul

No one knows you but you. We come into the world with loved ones staring at us full of love, and I believe when we leave this world, it will be the same on the other side. For now, I will embrace life and live in the now (of course with my red cape).

Why Tomorrow

Who cares? I'm here today…what shall I do? First, I'm grabbing that red cape. You cannot worry about what's not here. This is how we "Live in the Now" (another great book by Eckhart Tolle). I read this book years ago, before my divorce. When I became unhappy, I realized that I was living in the now, and he was living in the future—way into the future. I'm not saying you don't plan vacations, appointments, retirement, children, etc., but living should happen today.

My ex and I were about to change jobs and states for the first time in our lives. We were both in our early 30s. He looked at me one morning and said that we should go somewhere for two weeks before we started our new journey. We both had a lot of airline miles. I said right away, "Let's go to Greece." If you are going to use free miles why not go far away. It sounded intriguing. He agreed to let me plan this trip. His trips were always, planned out from a.m. to p.m. My trips…not so much. Nevertheless, Greece was an exciting trip from the beginning.

As we got off the first leg of our journey, the flight attendant asked us, the only Americans on this flight, to take care of this Greek lady that spoke no English. She appeared to be 99 years old and they were worried she would get lost and miss her flight. Now that I think of it, I'm sure she had dementia. What were we to say? This threw a monkey wrench into our plans to leave the airport by train and have a quick lunch in Germany. We decided to drag her along, hoping that no one thought we were kidnapping her. Only once did we lose her. I'm not sure to this day how we managed this but we made it to the next leg of our journey and kindly told the next flight attendant that we had to hurry off the plane in Athens.

We enjoyed Athens for two days. My ex asked me where we were headed to next. I looked at him with a big smile and said, I was thinking the islands. He was shocked that I had not planned anything beyond those two days. He panicked. Honestly, I had heard it was cheaper to travel when you were within a foreign country instead of making plans from the United States. Ends up, I was right. Still, he was not pleased but more concerned.

We ended up flying to Santorini where in mid-March it decided to snow. Yes, snow. Never in 100 years had it snowed in March until that year. We had swimsuits, appropriate spring clothes and a beautiful place to stay looking out over the Aegean Sea. The problem was we didn't have heat. None. After our first night cuddled up in a twin bed and still freezing, we had to move inland to the only hotel on the island that had heat. No view and it was packed. Did I say that this was the year that Atlanta was hosting the Olympics and we won that spot over Greece? They did not take kindly to us Americans. Try being Southern and changing your accent. Ha!

Our journey continued like this the entire trip thanks to my ex allowing me to plan, or not plan, our trip. I'll admit sometimes it was a bit unnerving, but we took it a few days at a time. It was one of the best trips of my life. Did I mention that was the only trip I ever totally planned myself with him?! Ha!

Every morning you get out of bed, just remember that YOU ARE ALIVE to see another day. Use it wisely, softly, lovingly. Find your laughter for the day, take those deep breathes, and go. Go into the day! (Did you even need that red cape today?)

Partner(ships)

Cancer is hard for partners, too, but stop—they don't have cancer so you tell them what you need as the victim. Besides my hugs, I have Ben run get my groceries, my coffee and rub my aching back. Okay, so maybe I take a little advantage, but he knows. ☺ Ben is a dream. Your turn. Don't let your partner take your red cape however, but it's okay to snuggle together when needed. Just always remember that your partner may need special attention at times too.

One of the things I love most about Ben is how he's always looking to make life choices healthier, easier. Ben is a forward thinker and has moved mountains to change communities to have healthier lives. When I asked him to read *Blue Zones, Lessons for Living Longer from the People Who've Lived the Longest* he devoured it in one long night. A week later he was on a plane sitting on the doorstep of the author, Dan Buettner. Dan was not interested in big corporations. However, Ben has a winning personality and is seriously the smartest man I know. He convinced Dan to listen to his idea to take this book and bring it to life in a big way to change lives.

I should have incorporated these ideas immediately. Why people live to be 100 and older in healthy bodies. These folks are still wearing their red capes without cancer. One guy even left the U.S. with his pending death, to go back to his home country in Ikaria, Greece to die. He ended up thriving and surviving in his home country. He later died, but not from cancer. This is radical remission.

To this day, they both continue to make a better world.

Wake up, America! We can all live in the Blue Zones here and now. Thanks Dan and thanks Ben for the partnership you developed and for continuing to make the world a healthier place.

This is why Ben believes that I can go into remission. There are days when I tell him I feel I am by myself trying to find the right path. He stops his busy life and sits down with me not only to calm me but to jump into my research, talk to a doctor and to always, always, give me a big hug. We are so alike and literally know what the other person is going to say or do. We have traveled so many places, thanks to his job and his many airline miles. The best part is neither one of us are planners so our trips are always an adventure. I need a new book to write just about our travels. It's amazing to have a partner so connected.

I know for a fact that Ben gets as nervous as me before my scan news. That's why I offer a gummy to calm him the night before. I am usually the one assuring him that night that everything will be good. You say this enough and it seems to be working. But it is still nerve racking.

Our partners are also in pain, and it is important to remember that they also need a big hug and reassurance…but don't give them your red cape.

C(ancer) Card

There are appropriate times to pull the C-card: store discounts, parking spaces, cutting the bathroom line, cutting the wait line at a restaurant, getting on the airplane first and when you need to cancel something. Never ever use it to get out of something. You may be jinxed. You deserve some kind of break and special attention so take it my friend. (Thanks again, Susan, for reminding me.)

We live in town in Nashville, on a street where there are few driveways and a lot of alleys. Unfortunately our alley behind our house has no room for our vehicles so I park right in front of our house. Mind you, the street is a public space and anyone can park anywhere. Just out of respect, you would think people would park in front of their own homes, however, we have a lot of "rented" homes that house too many young renters with boyfriends and girlfriends that visit quite often and add to the many cars parked out front. We have cameras and one points right to the spot in front of our home. What I consider *my* parking space. I became afraid to leave home in my car because when I returned to my space there might be a giant van there (next door boyfriend) that would stay for a week and I would be forced to park across the busy street. Worst of all, that van blocked our lovely view.

After a month of this, I took drastic steps. First, I called one of the next-door neighbors, and told her about my cancer and that I needed to park in front of my house. (Mind you, I walk three to six miles every day). I also told her that I would appreciate her assistance in informing everyone in that home and their visitors not to park in my spot. Feeling a bit guilty, I took them all appropriate gifts. It worked at first. But renters changed. Boyfriends changed. So then I took a more drastic approach.

I put on my red cape, sat down, and ordered an orange cone along with a handicap sign that slides over the top of the cone. My husband said I'm going straight to hell. I informed him that with

Stage IV cancer, I deserve some kind of special treatment and to me that included my damn parking space in front of my house. I keep it in the trunk of my car when it is parked. It has never failed me to date. So don't be afraid to play the cancer card.

PART XI: Courage to Heal

I'm leading you on a pathway to feeling better, feeling inspired, sharing courage, and knowing that there can be better news at your scans. Are you listening? If not, where is that damn red cape? Grab it right now.

Faith and Tears

Meditate, pray every day, and believe. This goes along with being grateful. Today you may be faced with chemo or radiation. Keep in mind that your immune system must be King and Queen and fed appropriately. Do not worry about tomorrow.

Today, be grateful that both Eastern and Western medicine has given you a potential way to rid yourself of cancer and/or possibly live longer. Have faith and believe it is working. Have faith that your researched medications and supplements (and healthy food) are working.

Stress can steal your faith. Stomp it out. Throw your red cape over it and say abracadabra. You cannot afford to let this now be a part of your journey. Not just your faith, stress will steal your thunder, your time, and your immune system. When it happens, exercise, meditate, read a fun book or watch a funny movie. Just stop it! Your red cape will remind you as it will not allow stress under the cape.

Trust me, I know there are those days that life seems or is, unfair. Those days when you ask yourself, can I really take all those supplements, can I face another day of chemo or radiation, can I find a way to get out of bed because mentally I'm drained? WAIT! Yes you can. Go ahead and cry those tears right now after these thoughts. Cry hard, and scream hard because cancer sucks and the cancer journey sucks, too. But it's what we have now. Most importantly, remind yourself that radical remission is possible. There will always be those moments when tears are necessary and a good scream is a must.

Someone once told me, God never gives you more than you can handle. Hmm…for now, with these thoughts, again have a little cry. The tears clear the eyes from all the muck of the day and night so go ahead and let them flow. Besides, when you feel emotional, it frees the soul.

Remember Jesus suffered and He never complained. He wore a robe, so He doesn't mind that you have a red cape.

Routine

Every single day I awake and say to Ben, even if he is still asleep, "Good morning, good morning." Routines might irritate your family, but eventually they'll come around and smile. The best part is YOU will awake with that red cape to start your day and your first thought should be "I am grateful I am alive." It's amazing how the attitude you take when you step out of bed will affect the rest of your day, with or without cancer.

At this point in your life, if you haven't already, make a weekly routine and try to stick with your schedule. It will motivate you, make sure you move more, work on healthy cooking more, read more, research more and be grateful. See where I am going with this? What are you waiting for? Go ahead, as NIKE says, and "just do it." (With your red cape, of course).

As I mentioned earlier, my daily morning routine starts with coffee and reading and then my daily walk or strength training. When I'm in Utah, it's playing pickle ball, e-biking or hiking. I do find time for weight lifting in my makeshift gym in my garage two times a week. You can set a clock to this routine. But then, what do you do with the rest of your day? My afternoons are unpredictable, but I always find time to nap.

Part of my routine is reading a good fiction book. Find a friend or two, pick two great books, read them, and then talk about them at lunch or dinner. This is much more fun than a huge book group. My sister is my book club, and she is a kickass reader all the while busy as a bee. I have learned to send her a book when I am at least six chapters in (and she still finishes first). I have no excuse except I think I have a short attention span. Our book club makes my day and becomes an inspiration for me. So I advise you to find a friend and some good books to read.

Funny Little Children

Bad day? YouTube funny children videos, FaceTime a niece or nephew (under age three), and just watch them play. What makes this even more humorous are the adults who may be interacting with them. Kids are so honest and pure it makes you wonder when did we adults lose our play? Well, some of us (me) choose not to grow up. Getting older…unfortunately, I can't stop that.

I honestly used to think I would never have children. I was busy trying to earn a lot of money and establish a career. I loved my nieces and nephews and thought this was enough for me. In fact, my mother sensed this and every family get-together (which is a lot when you are from the South), I was placed at a table with the children. There were five of them. At the time, I was in high school and they were all under the age of five. My mom thought she was so clever. She didn't realize that this was the highlight for me of our get-togethers. The adult table was arguing about something that didn't matter while we were laughing and being silly.

One such time when the adults were arguing a bit too much, I took my nieces and nephews on a car ride to look at Christmas lights. They were so excited. They thought I was the bomb. Seat belts were not a thing back then, so I jammed four in the back and one in the front with me. I drove a red hand-me-down '65 Mustang. (I had no idea the value of this car at the time.) Sure, we looked at all the beautiful Christmas lights, but more importantly, we did doughnuts in the cul-de-sac of a neighborhood until we were all crying with laughter as they tumbled around my car. Upon returning, I made them promise not to tell the adults. The first thing they did was tell the adults. Ha!

These nieces and nephews are now all grown and thriving. All but one has children, and the one who doesn't owns dogs that are their children. I respect that I really do. My niece was like me and no one thought she would get married nor have children. Well, well. She had Charlotte and this bright child lights up everyone's life. When she was nine months old, my sister (her grandmother) and I met in Chattanooga so I could spend the day with her. I took her to the aquarium and she loved it. We went back for a nap that didn't work. She only made my sister and I look like fools pretending to sleep. We caved.

Fast forward to her being two and a half, my sister took her to the Atlanta aquarium and she exclaimed, "Aunt Liz took me to one of these one time." No joke. She was talking in full sentences at sixteen months old. Everyone was amazed. That talking can be embarrassing too. Big reveal here. I have a problem when I am out walking that I need to go potty. The only problem is, there is never a potty, and interestingly enough, I don't mind going behind a tree or bush when there is one. Remember I was a runner.

I was on the beach in Kiawah doing my five mile walk when the urge happened. Of course I was on the phone with my sister who was keeping Charlotte. My sister bursts into laughter, especially when I told her I had to do my business behind the very thin seaweeds in front of beautiful homes, while on the phone with her. And of course she tells Charlotte. Fast forward a few days later at my Aunt's house in Atlanta where they were having a small family get together, one of my Aunts said, I need to go to the restroom and Charlotte burst out with "Aunt Liz pooped on the beach." Nothing is sacred with children.

Much like Charlotte, my own children brought such happiness and laughter to me as little children and even now. It was those nieces and nephews who secretly made me want to have my own one day. If you decide not to have children, dogs are great.

NOTE: Spend time with little children but don't give them your red cap.

You need it more right now.

Chill-in

Naps: Take them! Take them! Take them! I rarely miss nap-time. I recommend napping 30-45 minutes every day, under your red cape of course. You'll walk up refreshed and ready to have a fun evening. Your body finds healing power in sleep, even in those naps. Sometimes I sleep but sometimes I just meditate. It really is a time to chill, to have a blank mind and to let your soul be at peace.

Music is good for the soul and your mental state, too. Whether you play an instrument (even badly), do it! I have played at the piano for years. I used this talent to enter my local county beauty pageant in order to earn money for college. I was confident even though I wasn't the most beautiful. I won and this led to the Miss Georgia pageant and more college money. I didn't tell my family about the local pageant because I didn't want them to laugh if I lost. They were shocked and a bit mad especially when I was on the front page of the paper the next day. (I lived in a small town).

When we downsized after our children left for college, I had to sell my baby grand piano and for a few years, didn't have anything to play. About two years ago I bought a full-size keyboard and sometimes I just sit and bang on it to take my mind away. It never fails to shower me with music memories and peace

One terrible story with which God has forgiven me. I only hope the preacher's wife forgives her now 60 something year old son when she reads my book. I played the piano at our church for many services - mostly as a fill in. The preacher's son was my friend and his friend was my boyfriend. We would hang at their house in front of the little church. He was a fun bad boy and smoked pot. I decided to try it forgetting that I was playing that evening. We were just chill-in. Let me tell you, I could not stop playing verses—verses that weren't even on the page. I was so chilled. The music minister went along and just kept singing until I finally tired. I looked at our preacher's face and he just smiled and then gave the stink eye to his son. He would at times make him sit behind him in front of the entire church facing the congregation if he was upset with him, and this was one of those days. My fault. *Wait a minute, was it?* I was happy my family wasn't there that evening. Lesson learned.

No matter your taste, don that red cape. Chill and feel the healing.

I Love You

You are my family. This is our journey, our story, and we are not done. Inspire yourself as well as someone else to never ever give up. My friend, you've got this!

BELIEVE! BELIEVE! BELIEVE! I go into every scan with the faith and belief that I am healing. I ask for prayers every time because I know it takes a strong village. Two heads are better than one. You get where I'm going with this belief: God hears prayers and He hears yours. However, if you don't believe, God gives you this right, too, even though everyone else is praying for you.

I love you and all your supportive family and friends because I understand what it feels like to not only hear the words "you have cancer," but to live it every day.

Share the love.

Buy a friend a red cape

About the Author:

Liz Leedle, a Stage IV cancer warrior, lives in Nashville, Tennessee and part-time in St. George, Utah with her husband and two French bulldogs. Together they have two daughters on opposite sides of the U.S. one in California and one in DC, two sons who also live in the Nashville area, and one grandson. After 20+ years of fitness training and teaching Exercise Science courses at a local college, she is retired (mostly). Liz now spends her time doing all of the things she is inspiring you to do as a cancer warrior.

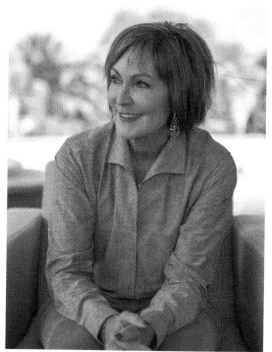

You can reach Liz at lizleedle@aol.com. Some things never change.